Where Does It Hurt?

About the author

Max Pemberton is a practising doctor. As well as a degree in medicine, he completed a degree in anthropology for which he was awarded a first and a prize for academic excellence. Max has worked in a broad range of medicine from A&E, geriatrics, adult psychiatry, surgery and paediatric palliative care. He is also a columnist for the *Daily Telegraph* and *Reader's Digest*. His first book, *Trust Me, I'm a Junior Doctor*, was a BBC Radio 4 Book of the Week.

Where Does It Hurt?

What the Junior Doctor did next

Max Pemberton

HODDER &
STOUGHTON

Author's Note

While everything that happens in this book is based on real events, the characters are composite characters and should be considered inventions of the author.

First published in Great Britain in 2009 by Hodder & Stoughton
An Hachette UK company

First published in paperback in 2009

1

A CIP catalogue record for this title is available from the British Library

ISBN 978 0 340 91992 7

Typeset in Rotis Serif by Hewer Text UK Ltd, Edinburgh
Printed and bound by Clays Ltd, St Ives plc

Hodder & Stoughton policy is to use papers that are natural, renewable
and recyclable products and made from wood grown in sustainable
forests. The logging and manufacturing processes are expected to
conform to the environmental regulations of the country of origin.

Hodder & Stoughton Ltd
338 Euston Road
London NW1 3BH

www.hodder.co.uk

To Ellie

Chapter 1

That man spat at me. It took a while for what had
happened to sink in. He definitely spat at me. The glob
of spittle sat on the pavement a few inches from my feet,
glistening. I wasn't sure what to do. No one had ever spat
at me before. And no one came to my rescue because I
wasn't on a ward, and the man who spat at me wasn't
a patient, just a random passer-by. I hadn't even looked
at him, let alone done something to provoke such an
attack. I decided to adopt my middle-class-and-suitably-
outraged look. Yes, that'd make him sorry. He didn't turn
round, though. Damn.

I turned to the man sitting next to me. 'Don't worry,'
he said. 'They're always doing that sort of thing.' He
slurped some soup from his polystyrene cup.

'But . . . but . . .' I began, but failed to find the words
to describe my indignation.

As I sat there, though, it dawned on me that the man
who had spat at me had done so because he'd thought
I was someone else. He hadn't realised I was a doctor,
sitting on the pavement trying to persuade a patient
with a gangrenous leg that he should come with me to
hospital. The brutal truth was that he thought he was

spitting at a homeless person. Had I really managed to blend into life on the street so quickly?

I looked down at myself: ill-fitting T-shirt, jeans, grubby trainers and a rucksack on my lap. Not so much George Clooney as Worzel Gummidge. I knew it had been a mistake not to wear a tie.

The man next to me was picking at a scab on the back of his hand now. He really did smell. I wondered if I should mention it, but thought better of it – I'd already been spat at once. This, I concluded, as commuters stepped over me, was not how things were supposed to be. I hadn't endured a year as a junior doctor, the plankton in the medical food chain, to sit on a cold pavement being spat at. I'd spent a year prodding and poking every orifice of the general public, and had thought I couldn't sink any lower. What had I been thinking when I'd agreed to take on this job? I thought back to earlier that day, the morning of my first day in my new job. It had started off so well . . .

It had been a bright, sunny morning. My flatmates, Ruby and Flora, were starting new jobs too. We sat and ate warm buttered crumpets while the sun streamed in through the window and we gaily perused the morning papers. Flora had made a pot of fresh coffee, which we drank leisurely around the kitchen table.

We were so relieved that our first year of junior-doctor hell was over and we could look forward to our budding medical careers blossoming in our chosen specialities. Sure, we were still junior, but now we were slightly more senior juniors. We were no longer

2

plankton, more a simple, multi-cellular organism that gets shouted at a bit but not so much as before. We were filled with excitement at the prospect of the day ahead. We wished each other luck as we left the flat and skipped off to our respective new jobs, whistling as we went.

OK, it didn't happen like that – I admit it. That morning was a bit of a blur. I remember waking up to screams of pure, unadulterated pandemonium as both Flora and Ruby realised they had overslept. 'You said you were going to wake me,' Ruby yelled, as she tried to clean her teeth and brush her hair at the same time.

'I did not! You said *you* were going to wake *me*!' yelled Flora, as she toppled into the ironing-board while she was trying to get a pair of tights on.

I opened one eye and saw the time. Fifteen minutes before I was supposed to start work. Oh, no. Ten minutes later I was running out of the door, having showered, dressed and smoked a cigarette. If you learn one thing as a junior doctor, it's how to get ready for work at lightning speed and still have time for a cigarette break.

I ran to the train station, joined the throng of commuters waiting on the platform and began to wake up properly. Another great skill you develop as a junior doctor – far more useful than how to save someone's life – is how to do nearly everything required of you while you're still half asleep and yet appear totally awake. The train slid into the station and the throng moved forward through the doors. Standing in the few square inches of space I had managed to claim as my own, I had time to think calmly about the day ahead – and do up my fly.

The intention, of course, had been to get an early night. But we'd just survived a whole year of abject misery so it was only fitting that we saw it off with a bang. And, boy, was that bang still going on in my head. My mouth was dry and my headache pounded to the motion of the train going over each sleeper.

Right. Time to focus. Get into doctor mode.

I wasn't sure why I'd taken this job. I'm sure part of it was nothing more than morbid curiosity – and, of course, it offered an escape from the wards, with their flickering electric lights, clipboard-wielding managers and barking consultants. But more than anything it was because I wanted answers. The city is littered with fragments of broken lives. We see them in shop doorways, asleep on park benches. We see used needles in the gutters and empty beer cans floating in the canal. Our lives and theirs run in tandem but rarely cross, but when I began work as a doctor people from all walks of life became my patients, which included those from the seedier side of life.

In fact, because sickness and disease are enmeshed in poverty, I saw a good deal of them. Throughout my first year, as I stood in A&E patching up the homeless, the alcoholics, the drug addicts and sending them on their way I asked myself again and again if I was I doing any good. Was I really helping them and, if not, how could I? I was given tantalising glimpses of their history as they shared strands of their lives with me, and wanted to know why the trajectory of their lives was so different from my own and why some people could cope and others couldn't. I longed to know the real stories behind the people we step over on our way to work, who pester us for money or mug us late at night. At what point in someone's life do they make the choices that result in them injecting heroin, say?

'Oh, you're such a freak,' said Ruby, when I first explained the job I'd applied for. 'Why can't you just be like everyone else and get a normal job looking after normal people?' We had been standing in A&E, and at that point someone had walked in with a toilet seat stuck on their head. 'Well, you know what I mean. Normal for the general public,' she said, as the man tried to negotiate his way into a cubicle. 'No one actually works with prostitutes and drug addicts out of choice. Didn't you learn anything at medical school? The Holy Grail is nice old ladies who buy you Quality Street.'

This, I felt, was a little rich coming from Ruby. Her new job was working in trauma and orthopaedics. Surely the very name was enough to put off sensible people. She was paid to run to the scene of an emergency while everyone in their right mind was running away from it.

Flora had been a little more supportive. 'Well, I think it's a very interesting area and I'm sure it'll be rewarding,' she said, 'but if anyone gives you chocolates, don't eat them. They'll probably be laced with heroin. They do that, you know, to get you addicted. My mum told me.'

Although I didn't say it to Flora – more because her pager went off and she had to examine someone's rectum rather than the desire not to criticise her mum – this was precisely why I wanted the job. Everyone, from the person sitting in their semi-detached watching *EastEnders* to politicians debating in the House of Commons, has an opinion about drug addicts and the homeless. Some think they deserve our sympathy, others that they deserve a kick up the backside. I confess I didn't know what I thought, but I concluded that there was only one way to find out, and if you wanted to explore the depths to which humans are capable of sinking you wouldn't succeed unless you at least dipped your toes in the murky waters. I wanted to change my perspective, alter my view and see things afresh. Or perhaps Ruby was right and I had gone insane. Perhaps I was living proof that it wasn't possible to live on a diet purchased solely from a twenty-four-hour garage and retain your full cognitive abilities.

The thought continued to niggle as the train drew up at my stop. While I was at medical school, I also did a degree in anthropology and became fascinated by the fact that society is not one homogeneous group: it's made up of countless sub-groups, whose members move fluidly between them. Here in the train carriage there was a mix of people from different walks of life, with different understandings of the world, existing in the same culture, yet two people standing next to each other might share little in common. While you can explore foreign lands and study their indigenous populations, within our own society there are layers of different cultures, pockets of people who are connected with other pockets, who are in turn connected to others, creating a web. The people I was about to start working with are part of society and I wanted to understand their world – to become an anthropologist in my own city. Was society to blame for their failings, or were they to blame for society's?

To the horror of my friends and family I had taken a job working in a homeless outreach project, and a clinic for drug addicts. 'Project', 'clinic': words like that sound reassuring, don't they? But the people who were going to be my patients would be bums, down-and-outs, drug addicts, prostitutes, rent-boys, pimps, the homeless, drunks, runaways, crack-heads, thieves and muggers. For the next year I would be their doctor. The rule of the job was that, as they wouldn't come to me I had to go to them. And, besides, if I wanted to try and understand their world, I'd have to join them in it.

The term 'outreach' is a misnomer: it's not so much a reaching out as a reaching in. Inside the city, right to the bottom. 'Reaching out' implies that they are on the edge of civilisation, but they are at its very centre, in the middle of the city, their lives are being played out in dank alleys and leafy public squares. They are everywhere among us, if only we look.

The train came to an abrupt stop and I was jolted back to reality. The doors opened, the throng of people pushed and I stepped off the train and onto the platform.

I walked out of the station into the morning sun, with crowds of commuters swimming round me, like shoals of fish. They pushed and jostled, clutching briefcases and lattes in steadfast determination, oblivious to those around them. I moved towards a doorway to avoid the crush and spent a few minutes scrabbling in my pocket to find a hastily drawn map. It was already nine thirty and I was late. I was not alone in the doorway. 'Spare any change, mate?' said a man sitting on the floor. I looked at him and paused, then shook my head. He looked at me silently, then caught the eye of another passer-by before repeating his request.

I stepped back on to the pavement and negotiated my way past streams of people trying to get to work. As I walked away from the station, the crowds gradually fell away, until I was walking down a stretch of road on my own. After five minutes, the shops began to look shabby with bags of rubbish lying uncollected in doorways, the contents spilling out. Paintwork peeled. Slowly urban decay began to creep in; the steady rot of neglect. The signs in the shops no longer catered for commuter affluence but cut-price telephone calls to Africa, laptops at knock-down prices and cheap clothing. The last two shops offered nothing at all, their smoky windows now decorated with posters and graffiti.

I checked the directions again and peered at the map. I was lost, surely. Further down the road I could see blocks of council flats, grey and forbidding. I turned my back and retraced my steps. Two men across the road stood motionless, watching me. I began to feel uneasy. Please don't mug me before I've even started. At least let me get a cup of tea first. They appeared to be communicating with each other without actually talking. One looked at the other and nodded, then crossed the road. As he was about to pass me he lifted his gaze from the pavement and said, in a thin, almost inaudible whisper, 'Brown or white?'

By the time I had registered this, he was already a few paces behind me. I stopped and turned. 'Sorry?' I hadn't understood what he was asking or why. His pace slowed, but he didn't turn, just crossed back over the road and resumed his position next to the other man. They stood for a few moments, staring at me with suspicion, then turned on their heels and walked in opposite directions. When I looked again they had vanished. I decided I needed to find my new office – quickly.

I glanced back at the shops and began to count the street numbers. There, nestled between 267 and 269, was a door. It had no number, no identifying features. To the left there was an intercom and a handwritten sticker: 'Phoenix Project'. This was what I had been looking for. I pressed the buzzer and heard a click as the door was unlocked. I pushed it open and went inside. It slammed behind me and I stood in front of yet another door with an intercom. I reached forward to press the buzzer, but before I could, it was flung open.

'Are you the new doctor?' said the woman, as she tried to push a bicycle past me. I nodded and opened my mouth to speak. 'Great. Come with me. We've got loads to do today,' she continued, without giving me chance to reply. She had beads round her neck and long flowing hair. I bet she's got a henna tattoo and eats organic rocket, I thought. 'I'm Lynne. You'll want to take that off for a start,' she said, looking at my tie.

'What's wrong with it?' I asked.

She didn't answer and barely looked at me as she attempted to negotiate her bicycle through the doorway and out on to the street. 'We've got to go to a hostel and review a man who's sick. Did you bring a stethoscope? Because we haven't got one here. You haven't got a bike? Well, you'll have to get the bus. The address is on this piece of paper. I'll see you there, OK?' She sped away before I'd had a chance to introduce myself. I crossed the road and stood at the bus stop, wondering if it was too late to get back on the train and find a job as a GP in a leafy suburb.

Medicine is supposed to provide answers. It assumes that, by following certain principles and theories, even complex constellations of symptoms can be rationalised and understood. The body is a machine and can be fixed with the right bit of tinkering. That's the theory, anyway. The reality is, of course, rather different. Doctors, while they sometimes might like to think otherwise, don't know it all. The medical model is not infallible. In fact, the more you understand of it, the more you realise we don't know very much at all. But there is still a common perception that when something's going wrong, a doctor will be able to sort it out. Which was why, after I'd met Lynne at the address she had given me, I found myself standing at the entrance to an old Victorian workhouse surrounded by a collection of men who wouldn't have been out of place in a Dickens novel.

'You the doctor?' asked one of them.

I hesitated. Was he going to show me his in-growing toenail? I wondered, as I noticed that he was not wearing shoes. 'Erm, yes, I am,' I answered tentatively.

'I've been sent to meet you. You've got to come this way,' he said, rather menacingly, and beckoned Lynne and me to follow. The other assorted men walked behind us at a respectful distance.

Lynne seemed to be on first-name terms with most of them. 'This is . . .' She began to introduce me to someone who had no legs and a gaping hole where his left eye should have been, sitting on a home-made skateboard. 'Sorry, what did you say your name was?' she asked me.

'Er, Max,' I said absentmindedly, transfixed by the legless man as he stared up at me with his one eye. Why had he no legs? Why was he sitting on a skateboard? I mean, obviously he was sitting on a skateboard so he could get about, but why? Surely this was against some Health and Safety ruling. He needed a wheelchair, Stannah stair-lift and gainful employment in a community project that took him on outings to the seaside.

I smiled politely down at the man as he shook my hand. Don't mention the skateboard, don't mention the skateboard. There was an awkward silence. 'I like your . . . erm, skateboard,' I heard myself say, and was immediately horrified.

The man didn't seem bothered. 'Thanks, me and my mates made it ourselves. Beats being carried everywhere.' With that he skated off, pushing himself along the ground with his hands. The little wheels had clearly come from a supermarket trolley and spun round like beetles on their backs before they found purchase on the tiled floor.

I looked round at the group of men with us, then

at Lynne. Why did nobody else find the situation bizarre? I vowed to fill out a form about the man as soon as I got back to the office. There was bound to be one that covered this sort of thing. I'd get him a wheelchair and a glass eye whether he liked it or not.

This was a hostel for single homeless men. Although they might have been bachelors, none seemed particularly eligible. A visit from a doctor was viewed as rather an event, and so I was escorted by a random assortment of men, unwashed and unloved, all hoping that somehow I'd be able to help them. On the scale of housing, Lynne explained, in a whisper, it was about as low as you could get without actually sleeping on the streets. Everyone wanted to be introduced to me, as though I were some visiting dignitary. Several of them did a little bow when I shook their hands and I was so embarrassed I almost started laughing. 'Sorry, I haven't had a shave,' said one man as I shook his hand. I looked down and saw that his hand was black with grime.

Single homeless men make up the largest group of people sleeping rough, and they are also the group for whom the least resources are available. This place offered the basics. There were no carpets, the old Victorian cornicing was dusty and the paint was peeling. I'd never been in a place like it before and it wasn't the sort of place you'd go to unless you had a very good reason, and even then I suspect you might try to find something else to do. Cities yield up their secrets slowly, and although I'd thought I knew the area fairly well, I obviously only knew a certain side of it. I used to live within a few hundred yards, shopped regularly round the corner, and my favourite restaurant is only a few minutes' walk away, yet I'd had no idea that this place existed. I must have walked past it a hundred times.

I was introduced to Warren the Warden, a Pickwickian, avuncular character whose proportions contrasted against the thin and weak-looking man he stood next to. 'This is Danny,' he said, while Danny hacked and coughed and spluttered. I hunched over him in his tiny prison-cell of a room, with the thin, sheetless mattress and bars on the windows, and listened to his chest. He'd been coughing up blood for the past few weeks. He also clearly had a mental illness. I suspected he had TB, an illness rife among the homeless. I explained what I thought was wrong, and was asked what we should do for Danny. The answer was simple: he needed to be admitted to hospital for treatment.

Danny's situation prompted more questions. At this point I had no idea how best to help him and others in similar situations. Often when we look for answers, we want to find someone to blame – the government, society, even the individuals who find themselves in places like that. But surely things aren't that simple. It isn't just about money, or wrong choices people have made, drugs or upbringing. I felt utterly impotent and overwhelmed by the desperation that surrounded me. Over a hundred years ago the hostel had housed the same groups of people it houses now. Nothing has really changed.

The men in the corridor looked at me expectantly. I

didn't have the answers to their problems so I walked out and back into the bustling city.

'And I'm Joy,' said the woman, scowling at me. 'I don't want no grief off you, yeah? You want your typing done you better be nice to me or I ain't doing nothing for you, Mister, you understand me?'

I adopted a fixed smile which I beamed back at her. Clearly her parents' wishful thinking when they gave her that name hadn't paid off.

'And look at what he's wearing. What you think this is? Savile Row or something? I tell you, you better stop with all that dressing-up malarkey,' she continued.

I looked down at myself. I'm not usually criticised for being too smart – quite the opposite. I tend to grab whatever I can and put it on in whatever order. I consider matching socks quite an event.

'They're going to eat you alive out there, looking like that,' Joy concluded.

'Here, change into this,' interjected Kevin, one of the nurses. He tossed over a carrier-bag containing clothes.

'Oh, thanks,' I said, as I tentatively peered into it.

Kevin seemed to understand what I was thinking. 'We always keep a spare stash of clothes for patients in case they need it so, no, I'm not sure if they've all been washed, but they'll do for today.'

I begged to differ. I didn't want to wear someone else's dirty clothes for a minute, let alone the rest of the day.

The office seemed to go quiet. Everyone stared at me expectantly. I looked at Kevin, standing there relaxed in his T-shirt and jeans. This, I thought, is my first test.

'Our patients tend to find a shirt and tie a bit

intimidating,' said Haley, another nurse, by way of
encouragement.

But do they want a doctor with scabies? I thought. I
pulled out a T-shirt. It had mud on it and was yellow
under the armpits. Was it my imagination or did it
smell of dead people? 'Fine. Thanks. I'll just go and
change,' I said, swallowing.

On my way to the toilets I met one of the patients.
He had a beard and wild, matted hair with little glasses
perched on the end of his nose. 'Hello, there,' he said,
in a surprisingly plummy voice. 'Are you our new
doctor?'

I smiled and introduced myself.

'Well, I expect you've heard that the last two didn't
make it past the first week. I hope you're going to fare
better,' he said.

'Oh, erm, no I didn't know that,' I replied.

'This job isn't for everyone, really. It takes a certain
getting used to. People feel intimidated by the patients,
find the environment challenging. And don't listen to
Joy – she likes to project this hard, ghetto persona but
she was born in Tunbridge Wells and collects china
cats really.' Between each sentence he took a sudden,
audible gasp of breath and paused before he continued.

'Right, OK, well thanks,' I said, rather surprised that
a homeless man should be so familiar with the inner
workings of the team. 'I'll see you around, no doubt.'

'No doubt,' he chirped, as he made his way up the
stairs.

I got changed into my new – or, rather, very old –
clothes and looked in the mirror. I was the antithesis,
no doubt, of how Ruby looked right now, dressed in

sterile surgical scrubs. I made my way back up to the office and was surprised to see the homeless man sitting on the desk chatting away to Kevin and Joy. 'You haven't been giving our new young doctor a hard time, now, have you?' he asked, and Joy fluttered her eyelashes.

'Now, would I do a thing like that, darling?' she said, raising an eyebrow at me. 'He knows who he's got to look after, don't you, dear?'

'Have you met Professor Pierce, our consultant?' interrupted Kevin, pointing to the homeless man.

I looked past the figure he was pointing to, expecting a consultant to materialise. None did.

'Yes, we met on the stairs a few minutes ago,' he replied.

I don't want *that* as my consultant, I thought, horrified. I want a proper consultant. Someone who's aloof and plays golf.

Before the conversation could progress any further, Lynne entered the office and handed me a piece of paper. 'We've had a referral. Would you mind going? It's just that I've got patients to see this afternoon and no one else is free.'

I looked down at the referral. 'Man seen looking unwell outside NatWest bank. May need urgent medical attention – possible problem with foot. Wearing dark blue sweater and green coat.' I turned it over, expecting more information. It was blank. 'Sorry,' I said, as Lynne began to walk away, 'is that it?'

'Yes,' she replied, smiling.

'What about a name? Date of birth? Address?' I flinched as I said the last word. OK, so he won't have an address, but a name – for goodness' sake at least give me a name.

'Nope,' replied Lynne. 'That's it.'

I'd thought I was a doctor, not Sherlock Holmes. How was I supposed to find him in an enormous city with just that description to go on? 'Where's the NatWest?' I asked.

Lynne shrugged. 'Don't know which one and, even so, there's no guarantee he'll be there. He was spotted by someone from the council's homeless team but they didn't get any more details. The best thing to do is start off back up the street and ask the guys that hang out by the station if it rings any bells. Failing that, ask them where Barry is, then find Barry and ask him. He knows everyone.' And with that, she left me clutching the most ridiculous referral I had ever been given.

I picked up my rucksack and headed downstairs. 'Good luck,' cried Joy. I detected the strong aroma of sarcasm. Or maybe it was the smell of mould from my T-shirt.

I walked back up the road until I came to the station. I stood there and looked around. This was ludicrous. Utterly ludicrous. I had to find a group of men who would direct me to someone called Barry, who would be able to locate a man with a bad foot last seen outside a bank. This would never make it into a script for *ER*.

I decided to get a coffee and reassess the situation.

As I queued up at the kiosk, I heard a voice: 'Hello, Doctor.' I turned. There was no one behind me so I looked down, and the one-eyed, no-legged man from earlier that day was peering up at me from his skateboard and I tried to fix my stare on his one good eye. 'You alright?' he asked. 'It's Talcott, I met you at the hostel this morning,' he said.

I saw my opportunity. 'I'm looking for a group of men that hang around the station,' I told him.

He sat in contemplation for a moment. 'I'm quite hungry, you know, Doctor.' A muffin seemed a reasonable price to pay for information, so I bought one with my coffee and gave it to him. 'Oh, yeah, I know who you want.' With that he sped off, zigzagging in and out of the pedestrians. I followed him to the back of the station, then into an alleyway, and was confronted with three men standing motionless staring at me and Talcott. 'Hi, guys, this is the new doctor. He's looking for someone,' and with that, Talcott sped off.

I suddenly felt very alone. I wasn't sure what the men were doing there, but I imagined it wasn't swapping knitting patterns. They eyed me suspiciously.

'You ain't nothing to do with the cops, are you?' said one of them.

'No,' I said, as emphatically as possible, giving a little snort for good measure but which came out more like a squeal. 'Lynne sent me. I'm trying to find someone,' I said, handing over my referral.

'Ah, Lynne.' They visibly relaxed. One of the men produced a piece of foil from behind his back. Aha! I've seen *Trainspotting*, I thought. You're doing drugs! I resisted the temptation to say this though. 'She said Barry might be able to help me,' I began.

'Oh, yeah, I've not seen him in a while. He don't

hang around with us when we do white. We can help you, though. I know who this bloke is.'

There was that word 'white' again. Obviously it was something to do with drugs.

'I saw him this morning. He's in a bad way I reckon, Doc.' He led me to the corner of the street and pointed down a road. 'He was down there earlier. He's got a manky leg so I doubt he's gone far.'

I smiled and thanked him and he nodded his head. At least he hadn't knifed me and stolen my wallet.

Sure enough, after I'd walked for a few minutes, I came across a man slumped on the pavement. 'Hello?' I shouted. 'My name's Max, and I'm a doctor from the outreach team. I got a referral from someone saying you had a bad leg.'

'Piss off,' he replied.

This, I thought, is going to be a long afternoon. I sat down next to him. A woman from the offices next door came out and gave him a cup of soup. She looked at me. 'I'm a doctor,' I said and she looked me up and down suspiciously.

'Well, he needs one if you ask me. He's been lying out here all day.' She went back in.

And that was how I came to be sitting on the pavement getting spat at. 'I got a kicking at the weekend,' said the man, while I was still reeling from the indignity of being mistaken for a bum. 'They're always doing it. I'm an easy target, what with my leg.' Technically it was dead from the knee down and beginning to rot. This, I concluded, was where the smell was coming from. 'Sometimes they spit, sometimes they just shout at you. Other times it gets nasty and they duff you up,' he explained, while continuing to drink his soup. He rolled up his sleeves and showed me the cuts and bruises from where he was attacked a few days ago.

It would be easy to blame this sort of thing on louts and thugs, disaffected youth, but the man who had spat at me was wearing a suit, for God's sake. It shows you can't judge a book by its cover: while he'd mistaken me for a homeless person because I was sitting on the pavement, I'd assumed that, because he looked presentable, he was a decent bloke.

The man next to me, Samuel, eventually agreed to go into hospital so I tried to help him stand up. Across the road a boy was watching me struggle, and after a few minutes he sauntered over. He was wearing a baseball cap with the hood of his tracksuit top pulled up. I wasn't in the mood for any more trouble. But as he got nearer he called out, 'You wanna hand?' Together we helped the homeless man to his feet, and together we supported him until the ambulance arrived.

Chapter 2

'You do know what the young ones call her, don't you?' said my patient, Molly, cackling. I shook my head. 'Cattle Prod, though don't ever say that to her face. Not unless you want to be taking your food through a straw for the rest of your life.'

I had already concluded, earlier that day, that Sister Stein – to call her by her proper name – was not to be messed with.

'Apparently, she came here as a bairn to escape the Nazis, though I'd like to have seen them try it on with her,' continued Molly. 'You know, she set this place up about forty years ago. She should have retired ages ago but rumour has it that if ever she leaves, the building will collapse.' Molly sucked her teeth and nestled down into the chair like a soothsayer. 'You got to hand it to her, she might be hard, but she's committed.' I wondered if, by the end of this job, I'd be committed – to an asylum.

Earlier that day I had begun in the drug-dependency clinic and had met the infamous Sister 'Cattle Prod' Stein. The clinic was technically in the same building as the Phoenix Project, but its entrance was round the corner. At the front was a large wrought-iron gate. It had creaked as I pulled it open that morning and I'd half expected to be greeted by a member of the Addams Family. Instead, there was just a short flight of stairs and, at the top, a security door.

I pressed the buzzer and a small, sturdy woman flung open the door. 'You're late!' she proclaimed, before turning on her heel and hobbling off through another door and down the corridor, impatiently dragging a walking-stick behind her as though it were a recalcitrant child. I looked at my watch. I was only five minutes late. 'I am Sister Stein,' she said, as I struggled to keep up. 'I am the lead nurse here at the drug-dependency unit.' Her slight Germanic accent, aloofness and short stature gave her the general air of a Dalek. 'I will show you round but you already have a patient waiting for you.'

There were two striking things about Sister Stein. First, she was old, in her late seventies at least. Second, and I suspect this was related to the first, she referred to herself, and everyone referred to her, as Sister Stein. Now, with the current fashion for 'assumed intimacy' in the health service and beyond, whereby everyone is either 'mate', 'dear' or at best called by their first name, this was rather a shock. I'd never come across a nurse who went by his or her surname and certainly never come across one who was called by her professional title 'sister'. I felt as if I'd stepped into an episode of *Dr Finlay's Casebook*, and was reminded of the good old days when doctors wore white coats and had their wicked way with nurses in the laundry cupboards – both of which have now been banned due to infection control. The term 'sister' is archaic, most having been replaced with 'modern matron', which just doesn't have the same ring.

When I had started work as a doctor, Martin, the modern matron in A&E, was constantly ridiculed when he was first promoted to the post. All together now: raised eyebrow, little finger to the side of the mouth, flare of the nostrils and a loud squeal of 'Maaaatron,' every time he walked past. The more sophisticated members of staff would break out in spontaneous renditions of the title song from *Thoroughly Modern Millie* but replacing it with 'Thoroughly Modern Martin'. Last I heard he was selling used cars in Newport Pagnell.

Sister Stein hobbled up the stairs, the stick banging on each step. 'Here,' she said, pointing to a small room, 'is the computer that prints the prescriptions. The prescriptions are left in this tray for you to sign each morning.' She could make even the most banal things sound menacing. I glanced into the room and saw a pile of paper about a foot deep. Surely there couldn't be that many drug addicts. Through the window on the landing I could see into the office of the Phoenix Project. Joy was sitting at her desk, filing her nails. I waved but she didn't look up. It had come to something when Joy was a friendly face.

We went up a further flight of stairs to a large, open-plan office. 'This is Amy and this is Tony,' said Sister Stein. 'They are both nurses and the patients' key-workers.' Tony had been chewing as we walked in, but on seeing Sister Stein he had stopped. She went over to him. Although he was sitting down, he was still taller than her, so she looked up at him. 'You aren't chewing, are you?' she asked.

He closed his eyes tightly and swallowed. 'No,' he said. She continued to stare at him, and I wondered if she was going to make him sit on the naughty step. Instead, without taking her eyes off him, she lifted her stick and, using it like a snooker cue, pushed the opened packet of gum on his desk into the bin. 'Good,' she said, and left the room.

Amy rolled her eyes. I shrugged, smiling, and followed, as Tony rummaged through the wastepaper basket.

We traipsed back down the stairs and through more locked doors into Reception. A secretary and the office manager were separated from the patients' waiting area by yet another security door and a counter behind reinforced plate glass partitions. There was a notice tacked to the window which read 'Rudeness, intimidation or threats of violence will not be tolerated'. I wondered if that extended to Sister Stein.

'This is Meredith,' said Sister Stein, pointing to the secretary, 'and this is Bruce, the office manager.'

'Hello. I'm Max, the new doctor,' I said.

Bruce peered at me for a moment and said nothing. I was about to repeat myself, assuming he was hard of hearing, when suddenly he took a deep breath, put his hand on his chest and said, '"Trust not the physician; his antidotes are poison and he slays more than you rob."'

I blinked. What was I supposed to do with that, I wondered? '*Timon of Athens*, Act Four, scene three,' he said.

'Sorry?'

He tossed his head. 'Never apologise when the words of the Bard are spoken. Drink in his language like nectar, dear.'

'Just humour him,' said Meredith, from the other side of the room. 'He's a frustrated actor.'

'Frustrated?' began Bruce. 'I'll have you know I'm classically trained,' he boomed, projecting his voice through the toughened glass so that a patient in the waiting room, with a scab on his face, looked up. 'I do mainly local productions, these days, and give my services for free,' he added.

'Oh, amateur dramatics you mean?' I said.

He pursed his lips. 'There is nothing amateur about our dramatics. I once shared a stage with Wincey Willis.' He sat down and began to type.

Sister Stein was already out of the door and I followed her into the waiting room. She stopped and turned to the man sitting there. 'And what do you think you're doing turning up here after all this time?' she said, and struck the side of his chair with her stick.

Surely that was against some Health and Safety ruling. You can't go round haranguing people like that!

He jumped up and looked down at his shoes. 'Erm, like, sorry, Sister. I didn't wake up in time the past few days. I was hoping I'd be able to get my methadone script today.'

She rattled her stick against his chair again. 'You are always doing this, Mr Papworth; it is not good enough. We are not here for you to drop in on when you feel like it. You are not going to get your weekly script and will be put back on daily dispensing as from today until you can show us that you are reliable. Do you understand?'

He looked sheepish. 'Yes, Sister,' he said and sat down again. 'I thought you'd be pleased to see me,' he said, dejectedly.

She moved closer to him. 'You are not the prodigal son and there is no fattened calf for you here,' she said sternly.

'I'm vegetarian,' he replied.

Sister Stein ignored this. 'You'll have to wait here until I've finished showing the doctor round and then I'll see you.'

He appeared to be sulking but managed to nod and muttered under his breath.

'And no muttering under your breath. It's your own fault you're in this situation,' she added, as she walked away.

I stood in one of the interview rooms as Sister Stein showed me where the panic buttons were located. 'If they pull an offensive weapon on you, press this,' she explained. I wondered if people ever pulled inoffensive weapons – like a rubber chicken or a feather duster.

'What will happen to Mr Papworth outside?' I asked, wondering if Sister Stein's walking stick constituted an offensive weapon.

'Well, he had been coming every week to get a script for his methadone, which he takes to his local pharmacist. It saves him having to come here each day. But he is three days' late. He's probably been using heroin again so it's back on daily dispensing here in the clinic until he can prove he can be trusted.'

God, it was like being at school, though clearly a school with a *very* bad drugs problem.

We walked back out into the waiting room where an old lady was reading a magazine. That's sweet, I thought. Somebody's grandma has come with them.

'This is Molly, your first patient,' said Sister Stein, pointing to the old woman.

'Her?' I said, a little too loudly.

'All right there, Doc,' Molly said, giving me a wink. 'You ready for me now?' She stood up and, with my arm to steady her, we went into the interview room.

It was comfortable, but the bars on the windows and the panic buttons lent it a sinister air. 'You're here to start treatment for heroin addiction?' I asked as we sat down. 'And you're . . . erm, eighty years old,' I said as I looked through her notes. 'So you're retired. What did you used to do?'

'Well, I worked as a hooker but . . .' she coughed violently '. . . I ain't done that in a while, obviously.'

I looked at her, bemused.

'I'm practically a frickin' nun these days,' she continued. 'I used to enjoy my work, I won't pretend I didn't. I cared about the boys that used to visit me – that's why they kept comin' back. I even used to darn their socks if they hadn't used up all their time.'

A tart with a heart, I thought. Well, more of a tart with a heart-valve replacement.

'Anyway, here I am natterin' on at you, Doc. I expect you got other junkies to see, ain't you?' She stared at me expectantly.

'Erm, well yes,' I said, then corrected myself. 'Well, no, not junkies. We don't call them that. They're people who have substance-misuse problems.'

27

She guffawed. 'Oh, don't give me that bullshit. We're all junkies. You can use whatever fancy words you like, it's all the same. No one gives a bollocks what you call them. We know what we are and if we didn't like it we wouldn't shove junk into our veins every day, would we?'

'OK. Well, you're my first patient so you'll have to bear with me,' I said, as I riffled through the reams of forms I had to complete for each new patient.

'Oh, it's easy,' she said. 'You go through that list of questions you gotta ask me, I'll say I wanna give up, you tick the boxes, give me the methadone, and when I get bored I'll start shooting up again.' She sat back and smiled widely, showing a row of dentures with bright pink artificial gums.

There was something rather scary and unpredictable about Molly: she was so straight talking that she managed to circumvent social convention. 'Well,' I began, reading through the form, 'when did you first start taking heroin?'

She sighed. 'Long before you were even a twinkle in your daddy's eye, son. Ain't you read my notes?' I confessed I hadn't, although I remembered seeing a large pile of notes on my desk that morning. 'Recently I've been using about two bags of heroin a day,' she said.

I wrote this down in the little box provided. 'A bag?' I asked, not sure how much this was. Were we talking clutch or tote?

'It comes in little wraps of cling-film, about the size of a fifty-pence piece. They call it a bag.'

It seemed strange that such a small amount could cause so many problems. 'Anything else?' I asked.

'Oooh, and a bit of crack too, when I can get my hands on it,' she said, as though crack cocaine was a special treat, like sirloin steak.

'Anything else?' I asked.

'Ain't that enough? Give us a break. How many grannies do you know on smack, for God's sake?'

I had to confess that I didn't know any. The nearest my own gran had ever come to drug abuse was when she'd taken two Lemsips in one afternoon. 'Do you drink alcohol?' I asked, my pen hovering over the next box.

'Oh, no, never touch the stuff. Rots the liver. You should know that, what with being a doctor.' Of course. Silly me.

I came to the next question: 'How do you fund your drug habit?'

She looked at me silently, presumably because the answer was self-evident, yet it evaded me. 'Well, it ain't on my effin' pension, is it? That barely even covers my rent,' she said loudly. 'All the bastard government gives me is a free TV licence. I'd rather get stoned off my face than watch the drivel on TV.'

I suspected that large swathes of the country would sympathise with her on this point, and suppressed a smile.

She explained that she augmented her meagre pension by working as a drugs mule. The local dealers paid her in bags of heroin for moving their stock. She transported it all over the city in her shopping trolley. 'Aren't you worried about getting caught?' I asked.

She raised her eyes to the ceiling. 'What policeman's gonna frisk an old lady outside Morrison's, for Christ's sake? But since I've knackered my hip it's not so easy carting the stuff around. I can't make my drops so easily. Thought I'd have another go at this place. It's been ages since I've been here and although you're a bunch of bastards it's more fun than the drop-in centre where the highlight of the day is bingo.' I wondered how bad a game of bingo could be that a drugs unit was preferable.

The form was long and after detailing the person's drug use it went into minute detail about the person's life: childhood, schooling, education, housing, family, past medical history, past psychiatric history, previous episodes in treatment, medication the person was taking, and so on. Every new patient, or patient returning to treatment after they had not attended for more than three months, had to have one of these assessment forms completed before they could start on a treatment programme. I flicked through the pages and sighed.

'Oh, don't worry,' Molly said. 'I've had that done loads of times. You can just copy it from the previous forms. Not much has changed, except I'm now on the local residents' committee. And my grandkids are older.'

'Do they take drugs?' I asked warily.

'No way. If I caught them doing that I'd break their necks – and they know it. Besides, no one round here would dare deal to them cos they know I'd be after them if they did,' she said, cocking her head and glaring at me.

While she seemed frail, I didn't doubt that she would strike fear into the heart of even the hardest drug-dealers. Like Supergran, but on crack. And although, for her, drug use was normal, it wasn't the life she'd choose for her grandchildren. She could change, too, yet she had admitted that when she felt like it, she'd go back to using and drop out of treatment. She was accepting failure before she'd started. 'So you're telling me you want maintenance, rather than to stop using altogether?' This was important: Molly's answer would determine the type of treatment I offered. It was the one bit of the job I felt confident about as we'd covered it in medical school.

In essence, two medications are available to prescribe for people addicted to heroin. The first is methadone, a bright green or blue liquid in the same class of drugs as heroin and morphine – the opiates. You take it every day as a substitute for heroin and it stops the physical cravings. Because it's prescribed the dose is accurate, and can be increased if you need more to stop the cravings, or brought down over several months if you want to get off it altogether without the unpleasant withdrawal symptoms. The downside is that to start with you have to come every day to the clinic to have it, and for safety reasons can only have a weekly or fortnightly prescription once you've proved, through urine tests, that you're not using heroin on top. Methadone doesn't give you a buzz like heroin does; it just stops the withdrawal symptoms. Given that most people use drugs for the buzz, this rather spoils the fun.

The second option is buprenorphine, or Subutex. This little tablet is placed under the tongue and dissolves slowly. It, too, is an opiate and substitute for heroin, but the dose can be decreased over weeks, rather than the months it takes with methadone, so users are detoxed far quicker. This is great if you're ready to be drug-free, not so good if you aren't. It works by blocking the receptors on the cells in the body which the heroin latches on to, thus providing the additional benefit of preventing any heroin you do take from working. It doesn't work if you're using more than a bag of heroin a day prior to starting on it. It's also incredibly expensive and reserved for people who are adamant that they want to be drug-free.

I'd assumed everyone coming into a drug clinic would want to be drug-free, but apparently not. 'Most of them will not give up,' Sister Stein had explained when she was showing me round. 'You will have a success rate of around five per cent a year.'

I was horrified. 'Is that it?' I asked.

'Oh, that's if you're lucky,' she replied. I looked round the waiting room, at the chairs, the posters on the walls, the administration staff, the nurses: all this effort, just for five per cent? 'But you're still thinking of abstinence, of getting people to stop,' she continued. I nodded. That was the point, surely. 'No. Maintenance. That's what you'll have to aim for with most of your patients. Just getting them to stop using heroin and keep taking methadone instead. That way they won't overdose and end up dead in some hole somewhere. If they're on methadone, they can get a job, pay their rent, get off benefits and finally give something back to society. That is the point of all this.' She struck the ground with her walking-stick several times for good measure. 'You'll have your work cut out just getting them to stop taking heroin, I can assure you,' she nodded and chuckled.

It seemed that Molly, despite being probably very easy to push over physically (which I wouldn't advocate, obviously), was not going to be an easy push-over when it came to convincing her to give up drugs. 'Look, son, I've been at this game for years. It's too late for me to change,' she said. 'You ask me if I could go back and do things different, course I would. I wouldn't choose to be a junkie, but at my age I've not got the energy to change. It might kill me? Big deal. So might my angina. At least with heroin it's gonna be fun.'

I wasn't convinced. She'd said she wouldn't choose to be a junkie, but she had. I began to write a prescription for her methadone. 'The starting dose is thirty milligrams and we can increase it slowly over the next week if you start to feel cravings, OK?' I said, as I signed the script.

'You need to watch yourself, Doc,' she said. 'They all know there's a new doctor startin' today. They'll see how far they can push you, so you gotta make sure you're firm wiv 'em.' Molly was full of such sage advice: clearly the stench of my naïvety had filled her nostrils the moment she had walked in. 'They'll try to get blues off you, especially cos you're new.'

'Blues?' I asked, suppressing the urge to ask if she meant rhythm-and-blues – even on my first day I knew it was unlikely that people would be trying to get CDs of Wilson Pickett out of me.

'Blues – Valium, you know, benzos.'

Of course. Valium, or diazepam to give it its

generic name. It was once the panacea for desperate housewives. The little blue tablets and their relatives in the benzodiazepine family of 'mother's little helpers' are highly addictive and now rarely prescribed. They produce a mild sense of euphoria and induce relaxation, so, explained Molly, are much coveted by people addicted to hard-core street drugs to use between hits. 'They're good for tiding you over until you can score some brown.'

I looked at her blankly. Why was everything colour-coded? It was like being at playschool – 'And in the blue corner, we have diazepam . . .'

'Heroin,' she translated patiently. 'It's called smack on the streets, or brown. Your smack-heads tend to be all right. They get a bad press but as long as they got enough for a bag or two they won't bother you.'

'And how much does a bag cost, these days?' I asked, as if I was comparing prices with those of years ago, like people do with milk or bread.

'Well, a bag will set you back a tenner, though most of it's cut with rubbish so it's not that pure.'

'And what's "white"?' I asked.

'Crack. That's the one to be careful of. Not physically hard to get off, like heroin, but, boy, it gives you such a buzz. You *can* get off it but you don't want to.' I nodded. 'You can get it everywhere, these days, but I remember when you couldn't get your hands on it for love or money.'

She gazed wistfully into the distance and I had to remind myself that she was talking about crack, not bananas during the Second World War. 'How much does it cost?' I asked.

'Well, a rock's about a tenner but you can get through anything from one a day to ten, depending on how you're feeling. It's very moreish.' Yes, just like Pringles. She'd only been sitting down for thirty minutes and she'd taught me more about drug addiction than I'd learnt in six years at medical school.

I spent the rest of the morning sitting on my own in a corner of the office signing methadone prescriptions. It was incredibly dull. Clearly, doing drugs was a lot more exciting than prescribing them. Several other patients had been booked in to see me, but none had turned up. I texted Flora, who now worked in a hospital down the road doing anaesthetics on the obstetric ward. 'Fancy lunch?'

She didn't reply.

Just as I was about to give up and face the humiliation of eating a sandwich on my own in the park, surrounded, no doubt, by a cohort of my patients in various stages of intoxication, she replied, 'Baby been delivered! Yes, pick me up in 5 mins.'

I collected the scripts together and put them into the tray marked 'signed', and made my way downstairs. In Reception, Tony was talking to Bruce. 'I'm going for lunch now,' I said.

'Yeah, so am I. I'll walk with you to the shops,' said Tony.

'"The welcome ever smiles, and farewell goes out sighing", *Troilus and Cressida*, Act Three, scene three,' said Bruce.

Tony looked at him blankly. 'I'm only going to get a panini, for God's sake.'

'Oh, get me a skinny latte, would you?' asked Bruce.

Tony and I left the building and walked down the road together. 'Why did you pick this job?' he asked.

I hesitated. 'I'm not sure. Out of curiosity, I guess.'

He laughed. 'You know what they say, "Curiosity killed the junior doctor."'

'Do they say that?' I asked.

'Well, no, but you're not a cat, so it wouldn't make sense.'

I wasn't sure that anything I'd seen or heard in the past two days made sense.

'You got any problems, come and see me. And don't worry about Sister Stein. She's all right. Her bark's worse than her bite. Though she's not a dog, so that doesn't make sense either.' I left him on the corner, still agonising over anthropomorphism.

Flora was bouncing around. 'Oh, I've had such a lovely morning. This woman came in and I did her epidural and helped with the Caesarean section and she hadn't decided on a name and after the baby was born she said she was going to call it after me! Isn't that brilliant?'

'Yeah, great.' I wondered if there were any comparable perks to my job, but the thought of a patient naming a bag of heroin after me, shortly before melting it on a spoon and injecting it into their veins wasn't quite the same.

'What did you do this morning, then?' she asked, before tucking into her sandwich.

I thought for a moment. 'I met an eighty-year-old drugs mule called Molly,' I began.

'Eighty?' interrupted Flora. 'And she's addicted

to heroin? That doesn't seem right. The only things eighty-year-olds are supposed to be addicted to are Murray Mints.'

'And I signed a lot of methadone scripts.'

'Have you got anyone off drugs yet?'

I laughed. 'No, I can confidently say I haven't.'

'Oh, well, you must,' continued Flora. 'A few babies on the neo-natal ward have been born addicted to heroin and it's horrible. Their mothers were addicts and now they're addicts. They're all limp and lifeless and they have to be given morphine in little droppers with their milk to stop them withdrawing. Can you pass the sugar?'

I handed her a few sachets. 'I'm having such a better time than last year,' continued Flora, in her jubilant stream-of-consciousness. 'The only good thing was that I lost two stone in weight. Would've been easier to do WeightWatchers, though.'

Back at the clinic, Bruce handed me my next patient's notes. 'Who is she?' I asked, as I flicked through the covering letter from her GP.

'"A maiden never bold, of spirit so still and quiet that her motion blush'd at herself,"' he replied.

I looked at him, then into the waiting room. 'You mean that girl sitting over there?' I asked.

'*Othello*, Act One, scene three,' he replied. I rolled my eyes and turned away.

'Are you Tammy?' I asked, as I walked towards the girl. She smiled. 'Yeah, that's me.'

'I'm Max, the doctor.' I led her to the interview room.

'You don't look old enough to be a doctor.' She giggled.

She didn't look old enough to be a heroin addict. 'Nah, I'm actually fifty-six. I just use good moisturiser,' I joked.

She was nineteen and very pretty, her tiny waist flaring into Rubenesque hips.

We sat down and went through the assessment form. She was injecting two bags of heroin and smoking two rocks of crack daily. That's a habit of £40 a day, I calculated, or £280 a week. 'And how do you fund your drug habit?' I asked.

'Prostitution,' she replied, then looked at her shoes.

'And what's your aim in coming here?' I asked.

'I want to stop being a prostitute. I've been doing it since I was fourteen and I hate it. I want to go to college and do something with my life. But I can't stop while I'm using drugs.' She sighed. 'That's why I'm here. I need to stop using.'

What she wants, I thought, is to be normal. Most nineteen-year-olds were going to college, thinking about their future, not injecting drugs in dark alleys. 'What about your parents?' I asked.

'Don't have any. I was in care.' She shrugged. She looked so street-wise, so mature, as she sat there, having already experienced so much of the world's harshness and brutality, but underlying that, she was vulnerable, scared and lonely. She desperately needed someone to lift her out of the quagmire into which she'd fallen. As I led her through to the dispensing room to get her first dose of methadone, I vowed she would be one of my five per cent.

That evening I sat at the kitchen table reading the newspaper and waiting for Flora and Ruby to return from work. I spoke to my mum on the phone. She was convinced that my new job signalled I was about to fall headlong into drug addiction myself. 'Are you sure no one offered you any drugs?' she asked repeatedly.

Honestly, if I hadn't considered them before, mind-altering substances were looking more and more appealing the longer I talked to her. There was also the inevitable medical query and today's hot topic was bunions. Did I think she had them and, if so, what could she do about them?

I told her I didn't know: my paranormal ability to visualise her feet from more than twenty miles away had been dampened by her incessant chatter.

'Stop being sarcastic and take your mother's ailments seriously,' she scolded. She went on to describe the angle of her big toe. I made the appropriate noises and continued to read the paper.

Eventually I heard the key in the latch and Ruby, then Flora, came in. Flora had a bottle of wine. 'Look what one of the fathers bought me to say thank you,' she said, holding it aloft. She rummaged in a drawer for the corkscrew.

'How was your day?' I asked, as Ruby sat down with a thud in the chair next to me.

'I'm so tired. There was a multiple pile-up and two drivers had to be cut out of their vehicles. One went into cardiac arrest and had to be transferred to theatre for us to operate on his ruptured spleen.' She was pale and tired but pleased with herself. 'I assisted in theatre and it took three hours to stop the bleeding. He arrested on the table twice but he pulled through in the end. It gives you such a thrill to save someone. Makes you feel like a proper doctor. Like it's all been worthwhile.'

There was silence for a few moments.

'How was your day? You saved anyone?' asked Ruby.

I thought of Tammy. 'Hope so,' I replied.

Chapter 3

Being God can't be easy.

'It's not,' Mr Allsop assured me. 'It's a lot of pressure. I mean, it's not something you'd want if you had a family.'

I tried to find a patch of ground next to him that looked relatively clean and sat down. Almost immediately I felt the unwelcome sensation of damp seeping through my jeans. I tried to ignore the fact that it hadn't been raining so God only knew what liquid I'd sat in, reposition myself and focus on the task in hand instead.

I'd found Mr Allsop sitting at the back of Tesco by the goods entrance where he had been living for the past few days. All his possessions were in plastic bags piled up in a trolley, which he pushed from place to place. I knew God was supposed to move in mysterious ways, but I hadn't expected to find him pushing a Tesco shopping trolley and eating an out-of-date pasty he'd found in a bin. Mr Allsop looked at me as I removed some orange peel I'd been sitting on, then added, 'Of course, I'm very blessed. I've got a whole host of heavenly angels to help me out.'

I'd never have thought of God being blessed but heavenly angels must indeed make the job a bit easier.

'The stress does get to me sometimes,' he continued wistfully.

While I'd only been in my job for a few weeks, I'd already become so accustomed to bizarre conversation that it hardly even registered as unusual.

'It's because of the stress that I had to come here. It's been nice to get away from all the responsibility that being the Creator of the universe brings.'

Of course, Mr Allsop wasn't sleeping outside the goods entrance of Tesco Metro as a respite from being God. If God exists, I find it hard to believe that he would be an elderly man in a tracksuit and trainers with a West Country accent sleeping rough. Although, to be fair, Mr Allsop had a white beard, so he got some points for effort. In fact, he looked more like Father Christmas than God, with his surprisingly clean white trainers resembling snow-covered boots from a distance and the red tracksuit setting off the festive scene nicely.

Mr Allsop had been mentally ill since he was eighteen. He was now in his late sixties. From the mountain of notes that had accumulated from his various admissions and now cluttered my desk at the Phoenix Project, it seemed that when he was younger his illness manifested itself in disturbing hallucinations and paranoid thoughts. But as the years went on, his psychosis had mellowed, and for the past few years he'd been steadfastly convinced that he was God. Usually he pottered along with his life, gently perplexed that he still lived on a council estate, rather than somewhere more divinely appropriate. Occasionally, for no discernible reason, he packed his belongings into plastic bags and headed for the streets. He frequented parks and train stations, slept in bus shelters and shop doorways. He also had a tendency to introduce schoolchildren to the Word of the Lord and hung around the gates to a nearby private school, giving stones to the bemused children and creating pandemonium among the parents, who thought he was a lunatic hell-bent on murdering their offspring. He was harmless but you don't pay to educate your child privately so that they can come face to face with mental illness on a daily basis. No, save that for the state schools.

During his periods of homelessness Mr Allsop would stop taking his medication, which made him worse. He became more evangelistic, convinced he must convert as many people as possible before he returned to being the divine saviour. Nobody wants an epiphany when they pop out for a packet of Munchies and a pint of milk, so the police had asked us to get involved.

A few months ago the situation had deteriorated when Mr Allsop thought that the packet soup in Sainsbury's (he has no brand loyalty – he's God, after all) contained lost souls: he went about opening them dutifully and emptying the contents onto the floor. Apparently the security guards found this a little bizarre so he was brought in to A&E by the police. From there he was admitted to a psychiatric ward, where he got markedly better. According to the notes, he was much more settled and his thoughts less disordered. This had been achieved by starting him back on the medication he'd previously been on, but had stopped taking. The cycle seemed hard to break: the periods of deliberate homelessness made him vulnerable to health problems and put him at the mercy of unscrupulous types who saw a man with all his possessions in plastic bags as easy pickings.

I didn't know what I could do to make this situation any better. It would be nice to think that all that was wrong with homeless people was that they lacked a home. But homelessness is often a symptom of a wider problem. The trajectory that had resulted in Mr Allsop sleeping rough was complex and multifaceted and as I sat with him I wondered what hope there was that I could interrupt it. I could get him into hospital, ensure his safety in the short term, but long term? Should I resign myself to the fact that this would continue indefinitely?

A shop assistant emerged from a side door and smiled at Mr Allsop. 'Hello, my child,' said Mr Allsop, and made the sign of the cross. Judging by his turban, I imagined that this wasn't the sort of blessing the young man was looking for.

He seemed undisturbed. 'Hello, Mr Lord,' he said, giving a little bow.

I stood up to introduce myself.

'Ah, good. I think Mr Lord will be needing your services very much. I tell him many times it is not good for a man of his age to stay here.'

'His name is Mr Allsop,' I said.

'No, no, he tell me his name is Lord. I know him very well. He comes here many times.'

I smiled to myself. 'Well, his name is Mr Allsop, but he likes to be known as Lord.'

'My name is Sohom and it is a pleasure to make your acquaintance, Doctor.'

Mr Allsop smiled benignly, then riffled through one of his bags and produced several items of food in various stages of consumption. 'Please, sir, you must not be eating these things. They will do you harm,' Sohom said, pointing to a packet of sandwiches. Mr Allsop understood this as a request for something to eat, and handed it to him.

Sohom hesitated, then took it graciously. 'There will be delivery soon so you must go. If my manager finds you here he will be very upset. You must do what your doctor says.' He bowed again to Mr Allsop, shook my hand and vanished back through the door whence he had come.

'I'm going to talk to some of my colleagues and I'll come back tomorrow, OK?' I said.

Mr Allsop nodded. 'Manna from heaven?' he asked, offering me a sandwich.

'No, thanks,' I replied. 'I've already eaten.'

I got back to the office, feeling overwhelmed by the enormity of his problems. Why couldn't things be nice and simple like on *Holby City*? Lynne and Professor Pierce, however, assured me that he needed admission and I welcomed their decisiveness.

'But what about longer term?' I asked. 'Can't we do something to stop him bouncing in and out of hospital?'

Lynne looked at me sympathetically, but before she could answer Joy interjected, 'Oh, you have so much to learn, darling.' She wagged a finger at me. 'When you find out how to keep all these people from the street, you sell that idea because it will make you rich.' She laughed. 'No, darling, actually you keep it to yourself because you'll make us all unemployed.' She cackled again and went back to her typing.

I wondered how Joy had got a job as a typist, given her proclivity for acrylic nails and her disdain for anything involving computers. I watched her for a few moments, transfixed by her ability to strike the keys with the pads of her fingers despite the jewel-encrusted talons attached to them and her lack of attention to what she was doing. Her interest lay solely in the machinations of the office social life.

'How many of them biscuits you gonna eat before you pass them over here, then, honey?' she shouted across the room to Kevin, who ignored her. 'You can't hear me? Or you just too rude to get off that fat backside of yours and come over here?' She got up and stalked over to Kevin, who was sitting at his computer, typing and listening to his Walkman, then grappled the packet of biscuits from him. I left them to it.

The following day I was sitting in McDonald's. Not out of choice, I assure you. I'd been there for more than an hour and, despite strenuous efforts, had already given in and eaten fries and a McFlurry. Now the vanilla milkshakes were looking tempting. I had to exercise some self-restraint if I was to remain this side of coronary heart disease by the end of this job.

That morning I had gone to find Mr Allsop but he was nowhere to be seen. I'd been to all the places I knew he frequented and there was no sign of him.

It had been frustratingly time-consuming; my list
of referrals was getting longer so I'd had to give up
and go to meet my next appointment. Working with
homeless people in the grottiest part of town took
me to some unusual places when I tried to track
down those who had been referred to me. Already I
had a working knowledge of landfill sites, disused
warehouses and graveyards.

Cities are filled with hidden places; nooks and
crannies that lend themselves to makeshift homes. I
had one patient who lived on a roundabout – I had to
dart through the traffic, stethoscope in hand, to see
him once a week. I couldn't be picky about where I met
them, and if they agreed to a meeting, it was on their
terms, hence my visit to McDonald's – it was a popular
choice with the patients. If it was up to me, knowing
that in return for meeting a doctor I was going to get
an all-expenses-paid meal at a restaurant of my choice,
I'm confident that McDonald's wouldn't be top of the
list. Actually, it wouldn't even feature on the list. But
Oliver had wanted to meet there, so I waited. And
waited. I suspected that this would be what the team
called a 'no-show': a self-explanatory term for a very
frustrating situation. Should I sit there and sample
the entire ninety-nine pence menu, in the hope that
at some point he might decide to turn up? Or should I
admit defeat and return to the office?

I'd had romantic ideas about the job before I started
it. I'd imagined myself roaming the streets, helping
the helpless. I suppose most doctors derive a certain
satisfaction from their patients' praise, so it's not easy
to be faced with a group who need more help than

most but are disinterested at best, and at worst abusive. OK, I'd never thought they'd be producing boxes of Cadbury's Roses for me, like patients on surgical wards, but I had at least thought that they'd be grateful. While people up and down the country were clamouring for appointments with doctors, I was trying to see patients who didn't want to see me.

At first, I was angry when people failed to turn up for an appointment, but sitting in McDonald's, day in, day out, waiting for people who might or might not turn up, I had to analyse my own motivation, and realised that the real problem wasn't with them but with me. While I hate to admit it, I had seen myself working with the Victorian 'deserving poor'. I'd imagined I'd be dealing with people down on their luck who wanted help. But this wasn't necessarily the case. To them I represented the authority figures they wanted to leave behind. I embodied the society that, for myriad reasons, they wanted to disengage from. They hadn't asked me to be there, so why should they have agreed to meet me when I asked to see them? And when they asked me for drugs that they could sell on the streets, I refused, when in their eyes, that was the only useful thing I could do for them.

Now I wondered about my desire to help Mr Allsop. Was it simply because I saw him as 'not normal'? I knew that I'd have hated to be him so I'd assumed he must hate being him. But what if he was happy in his world?

I was about to leave when Oliver walked up to me. 'You waited, then,' he said, by way of an introduction.

48

'Someone at the hostel was worried about you and asked me to see you.'

'All right,' he said. 'I'm gonna get something to eat.'

I stood up and walked to the counter to order him some food.

'It's all right,' he said indignantly. 'I got money.' He pulled out a five-pound note. 'What you having? My treat.' He smiled, and I ordered a vanilla milkshake.

I returned to the office to find a note from Joy on my desk. It was a message from Dr Whitfield, one of the consultants at the psychiatric hospital, who had phoned to inform me that Mr Allsop had been admitted. Great! One less job for me to do today. I gleefully crossed 'Get Mr Allsop sectioned' off my list, then glanced over the rest. If I ever lost it, whoever found it would be confused by its contents: 'Get sandwiches for Mark'; 'Find Waitrose bag-lady'; 'Has Chrissie had her leg removed yet?'

I phoned the ward where Mr Allsop had been admitted and the nurse who answered the phone explained what had happened. Last night he had been causing a nuisance in Tesco. Once again he had come to the conclusion that souls were being taken and hidden inside supermarket groceries by some malevolent force. It wasn't packet soup this time, but loaves of bread. He had ripped open Tesco's entire stock and emptied them onto the floor before Security was called. The police had carted him off to hospital where he had told the doctor who assessed him that he was sorry if Mr Tesco was upset, but he shouldn't go about stealing souls, should he? He had refused to come into hospital as a voluntary patient. As the assessing doctors unanimously agreed that he wasn't God and was probably suffering from a mental illness, he was sectioned under the Mental Health Act and brought into hospital against his will.

Thankfully, Mr Allsop was so used to the process that he hadn't resisted. 'In fact,' said the nurse, 'I think he quite likes the attention he gets here.' He had settled down on the ward and had been giving scripture lessons to the other patients, one of whom, the nurse told me, thought he'd been possessed by the Holy Spirit. 'All we need is Jesus to put in an appearance, and we'll be accommodating the Holy Trinity,' she said, with a giggle.

Ten days later Mr Allsop was ready to be discharged. The consultant who had been looking after him assured me that he was better, having started back on his medication. I wondered if this time he'd stay put in his flat. I walked onto the ward. Although I worked in the community (a euphemistic term for the dives I found myself in), the ward was an important part of the service. Many of the patients were too mentally unwell to remain on the streets and the best place for them was hospital. But sectioning could cause problems between the doctor who had initiated it and the patient. Many of the patients had serious physical problems, but they were usually willing to come onto the medical or surgical wards to have those dealt with. An overwhelming number of people on the streets have mental-health problems, for which they need treatment, but it is much more difficult to persuade them into a psychiatric ward.

A nurse escorted me to the ward office where I waited until Dr Whitfield, in the middle of a ward round, was ready to discuss Mr Allsop. A ward round on a psychiatric ward is different from that on a medical or surgical ward. It's more like a board meeting, but without the pie charts and mineral water. In fact, cups and glasses are banned in case irate patients use them as weapons against the doctors. The ward round takes place in the activities room, with the patient's ward nurse, the doctors, occupational therapists, psychologists, social workers, the patient, their family and, in fact, just about anyone who's involved in their care. Everyone sits in a large circle – like a séance, but no one holds hands.

While I waited, I looked at the list of patients on the whiteboard. I recognised at least three names as patients from the Phoenix Project. Oh, and Miss Nicholson. The last time I had seen her she was screaming that she wanted me dead. Great. I hoped she didn't know I was on the ward.

Someone banged on the door. 'I'm gonna kill you,' screamed Miss Nicholson. I reckon she knew I was there, and wasn't too pleased with me. It might have had something to do with the way she was screaming my name as she was dragged away by the nurses, or perhaps her parting shot: 'I'm gonna spoon his bloody eyes out.' Well, that's nice, isn't it? Despite the sudden need to use the loo, I decided to remain holed up where I was for the time being. I guessed I was off her Christmas card list.

When you're a doctor, no matter how stressful

or tiring it is, there's one thing that makes it all worthwhile – the feeling that, in a small way, you've helped someone. The added bonus of this is that they're grateful; they appreciate everything you've tried to do for them. In psychiatry, this never seems to happen, particularly with the really ill patients. There's no 'thank you', even though you're trying to act in their best interests. Instead they hate you. But the doctor-patient relationship really suffers at 'tribunals', the legal appeal hearings for those detained under the Mental Health Act – people who have been 'sectioned'. While a section means that we can detain patients against their will, and in some cases medicate them even if they don't want it, they can appeal against it. That's when the trouble starts. The last time I had been on that ward, I had attended Miss Nicholson's tribunal. I'd written the report outlining why we thought she should remain on section in hospital.

It was a burden to know that the report I would write for a hearing might result in somebody remaining on section, with their rights taken away. While it's ultimately the ward consultant's decision as to who should and should not be there, I had to write the report outlining the concerns of the community team when it came to an appeal. What makes it harder is that the patient reads what you write about them. Traditionally, young, up-and-coming lawyers cut their teeth at Mental Health Act tribunals. To be exact, they were cutting them on me.

'Can I put it to you . . .' begins the solicitor, at which point you know it's getting a little too *Perry Mason* and you'd like to slip back into *Casualty*.

The thing is, if you'd met Miss Nicholson, you'd have wanted her sectioned. Not only did she pose a risk to others, she posed one to herself. She was homeless, had drug and alcohol problems, and the fluctuations in her mood because of her mental illness meant that she'd tried to kill herself a number of times. I appreciate that it's important that decisions made by doctors are open to scrutiny but I'm not sure that these grand spectacles do the patient, let alone the doctor, any good.

People like Miss Nicholson, when they're very unwell, don't think they've got a mental illness. They don't think they should be detained or take medication. Of course she was ill. Of course she needed to stay in hospital, and as she wasn't going to stay voluntarily, she had to be on a section. I knew it, the members of the tribunal knew it and, most annoyingly, so did the solicitor. But I had to stand up and read out my report, accompanied by shouts of 'You little shit, I'm gonna get ya,' from Miss Nicholson, and then submit to an interrogation by Rumpole of the Bailey Junior, as if I was in the dock. I hadn't done anything wrong, except, maybe, take that job. It was just a big show, and all it had done was ensure that any relationship I'd built up with the patient was destroyed. The hearing adjourned, and when everyone returned, they had decided that Miss Nicholson should remain on the section.

'Well done,' said the solicitor as he left, as though it had been some competition from which I'd emerged victorious. The panel got up and walked out with the solicitor, leaving the nursing staff and me to face the aftermath of the hearing alone. And nobody, least of all Miss Nicholson, said thank you.

There was one problem: Mr Allsop was on high doses of medication, but he still thought he was God. The assembled professionals in the ward round nodded sagely. The art therapist showed us some promising paintings he'd done. I wasn't sure what they promised, given that they showed a lot of people burning in hell, but I decided to take her word for it. The general chatter was of how well Mr Allsop had done, how much better he'd got, far less evangelistic. Yet he remained utterly deluded and, unbelievably, Dr Whitfield thought he was ready for discharge.

'But he's not cured,' I said. Ruby was training to be a surgeon, working in trauma and orthopaedics. I couldn't imagine that she ever had conversations along the lines of 'Well, we haven't totally replaced your hip but it's a bit better and, hey, you can always hop.'

Dr Whitfield looked at me in the disconcertingly penetrating way of psychiatrists. I was always slightly on edge with him, worried that I might be giving away some dark secret I didn't know I had just by crossing my legs or something. He took a deep breath and let it out slowly. 'Why would I take away his delusion? That's all he's got,' he said, with a smile.

I began to protest, but then it dawned on me that he was right. Mr Allsop, free of his delusion, was just a sad, bumbling old man, with no family to look after him, no proper social network. Being God was all he had. He'd had a lonely life, dogged by mental illness. Who in their right mind would take away his one pleasure, his *raison d'être*? It didn't harm anyone, and it made him happy. Without his belief that he was God, what would become of him?

There was no guarantee that the delusions would go if his medication was increased but the side effects would get worse, encouraging him to stop taking it. And, faced with the harsh reality of who he really was, there was no telling what he might do to himself.

Mr Allsop was called into the ward round. He sat down and Dr Whitfield explained that everyone agreed he was ready for discharge. I told him I'd continue to see him at his home because I wanted to make sure he stayed there.

'Oh, yes, it's time for me to get back to my duties,' he said, and patted my leg. 'You've done very well. You might be in line for promotion to archangel now.'

'Well, that's very kind,' I said. He toddled off to pack, his world intact. He might be deluded, but perhaps he was blessed too.

Chapter 4

The woman in front of me snarled and looked away. 'Won't you just help me, for God's sake?' Kirsty snapped. She looked up at me, nostrils flaring, and scowled.

'Nobody but you can stop you taking drugs,' I said. I explained once again that we could give her medication to take away the cravings for heroin and stop the withdrawal symptoms, but it was up to her, and her alone, to stop using. She didn't speak for a few moments, and then she began to cry. It was often like this: they were angry at first, because they were angry with themselves. Then, for a moment, there was clarity and they saw how they were the architects of their own misery. Then they cried.

It had taken me a while to notice the pattern, but over the past month I'd seen so many drug addicts that I was beginning to see recurring themes. Medicine is all about pattern recognition. The basic theory underpinning western biomedicine is that bodies behave in remarkably similar ways. Constellations of signs and symptoms lead to diagnosis. It's not an infallible approach – there is always the quirky, unusual presentation, the unexpected, idiosyncratic manifestation of a disease or unexplained response to a medication or procedure. But by and large medical school is an extended lecture on how, when you strip everything away, we are all very similar. The trick for the doctor is to learn the patterns the body follows in health and disease and from this the diagnosis magically appears. It's rather like those Magic Eye pictures where you stare at what seems to be a wiggly pattern and suddenly see a great big rabbit holding a bunch of carrots (although there's always someone to contradict you and say it's the Empire State Building).

But the patterns I'd noticed, working with drug addicts, weren't just the things we were taught about at medical school. These patterns were not merely concerned with the physical way the body responded to addiction but the behavioural patterns of those who were addicted. For example, the ones who assured me, hand on heart, that they would stay clean this time, didn't. I'm sure that some do; it's just that I hadn't met them. 'This time, Doctor,' they would say, batting their eyelashes, 'I'm gonna get off the drugs for good.'

When I'd started the job I'd worried I might be too naïve as I readily believed their assurances that this time would be different. Now I was worrying that in just a short time I'd become cynical. I started them on methadone, they had their first dose, and I never saw them again. At first I thought they must have got lost or met with some misadventure on the way to their appointment.

'Don't be stupid,' said Sister Stein. 'You'll not see them again. They're too busy getting their next fix.'

'But they promised they were going to be clean this time,' I would remonstrate. 'They assured me.'

'Ha! The day that promises mean anything in this place is the day I shall eat my hat,' she replied. She often threatened to eat her hat. I'd never seen her wear one, perhaps because she said it so often and was sometimes proved wrong, she'd consumed them all.

I came to realise I was impotent in the face of my patients' addiction. I could plead with them, talk gently to them, be stern, but it was to no avail. All I could do was provide them with the resources to get off drugs, and it was up to them to quit. Part of me felt liberated by this: failure, by this criterion, was nothing to do with me. So what was I doing there?

Gradually I grasped that I wasn't battling mere physical addiction – in fact, that was the easy bit. Although I was prescribing medication to substitute for heroin, whole swathes of my patients kept using heroin on top. This was Kirsty's eighth time in treatment. The longest had been four months, the shortest a day. She'd never managed to give a clean, heroin-free urine sample. I flicked through her notes while she continued to scowl at me. I'd got good at being on the receiving end of scowls, but then again, with a sister like mine, I'd had years of practice.

Kirsty was twenty-eight and I'd met her in my first week at the drug-dependency unit and this was the fourth time I'd seen her. It wasn't the fourth appointment I'd given her – she'd had ten, but hadn't attended six: I suspected, from the urine-test results, that she'd been shooting up heroin instead. When it came to an appointment with me or shooting up, I was a poor second choice for Kirsty. I'd like to tell you that she had had a horrific upbringing, that she had run away from an abusive father, that she had fallen into drugs as an escape. It wouldn't be true. She had a fairly normal upbringing. Her mother was a hairdresser, her father worked in a local school as a caretaker. She had two older sisters; one was a legal secretary, the other worked in human resources for an electrical-goods retailer. None of her family did drugs. They didn't even smoke. Her parents had provided a stable, loving home life, with a caravan for regular holidays in Bognor Regis. OK, so this might be harrowing to some people, but it's hardly an explanation for hard-core drug use.

As I listened to each patient's life story I found myself constantly striving to find some connection between them and the others, some reason that they were set on this particular trajectory. Lots of them had suffered traumas, but by no means all. Anyway, many people suffer traumas in their lives and don't resort to drugs. What made one person choose this life while another just got on with things? If there was a pattern, it was obscured by so many other confounding factors as to make any conclusion meaningless.

'My mum and dad never wanted me,' said Kirsty, on the first day I met her. 'They were always saying I was a mistake. I knew it anyway. I could just tell.' She had had no contact with her parents for six years. The last time she had visited them, her father had told her to get out and not come back until she had stopped using drugs. She'd never been back.

'Don't you miss them?' I asked.

Kirsty stared at me blankly. 'Why?' she replied, with an air of wonder.

I was stumped for a response. Missing your parents when you haven't seen them in six years doesn't normally require justification. 'What about your sisters?'

Kirsty paused for a moment. 'Well, my older sister, she was all right. She used to look out for me when we were kids. Even when I stopped speaking to my family she used to send me cards and stuff, saying if I wanted to get clean she'd help. She even paid for me to go to private rehab for a few weeks.'

'What happened?'

'Well, you know what those private places are like. You pay them shedloads of money and they just sit round wringing their hands at you, telling you to stop doing drugs. They did my head in. When my sister found out I'd quit she stopped talking to me too.'

There was something about the callous, dismissive way in which Kirsty had met her sister's attempts to help her that infuriated me. I had this gnawing image of a sister, so desperate for Kirsty to stop using that she had paid vast sums, which perhaps she could ill afford, to try to help and had been met with contempt. There is a belief among addicts that residential rehab is the answer to all their problems. Patients often requested it. In the private sector they will happily take your money and provide you with a nice, peaceful room offering a view of rolling countryside, but in the state sector a residential placement is hard to come by. Unusually for the NHS, this isn't because of funding but because it isn't that effective.

At first this puzzled me. Surely it provided the time and space to get away from the temptations of the street, to battle the demons of addiction and win, returning clean and victorious. I mentioned this to Tony.

'You can take a horse to water but you can't make it drink,' he said. 'You can take the drugs out of the addict, but you can't take the addict out of the drugs. No, wait, that doesn't make sense, does it?'

I knew exactly what he meant. Removing the person from temptation doesn't address the underlying reason as to why they were using drugs.

'See it as a symptom,' explained Sister Stein. 'Drug addiction is not actually the enduring problem. It's the reason they take drugs that needs to be dealt with. It's a maladaptive coping strategy, a defence mechanism to life's problems.' This went some way to explaining why so many of the patients continued to use heroin even though they were on treatment to ensure they didn't have physical cravings. The methadone might stop withdrawal symptoms, but it didn't offer an alternative way to cope with the realities of life.

Heroin is physically highly addictive; crack is not. But both drugs are addictive because of the psychological benefits they provide for the user: the sudden rush, the euphoria, the overwhelming, all-enveloping sense of anaesthesia from one's life. It might sound heretical for me to say it, but if that's what you're looking for, then I'm afraid the drugs do work. If Kirsty was ever to succeed in giving up heroin she had to be prepared to endure life without her crutch. I could support her, but only she could make this decision.

Eventually she dried her eyes.

'I can increase your methadone this week if you think that might help?' I suggested.

She stared at me with dead eyes. 'Is that the best you can do? Just give me more of that muck?' Then the frown slid from her face. 'I did have some medication in the past that helped,' she said, smiling. 'A really nice doctor gave me some. I can't remember what it was called, though.' Now I felt profoundly uneasy. I knew where this was going. 'It was a little blue tablet. I think it was Valium.'

I remembered what Molly had told me on my first day in the job, and began to dread the argument that was about to ensue. I flicked through Kirsty's notes and could see that she'd never been prescribed any such thing by any of the doctors before me. She was trying her luck, I knew, but there was a brief moment in which I considered prescribing her a few weeks' worth just to avoid the battle. All that prescription would do, though, was treat my anxiety about her aggression. It would set a precedent, not just for her but for the countless other patients who would queue up outside, demanding the same treatment. Most importantly it wouldn't help her. It would give her another crutch, something else to become addicted to.

'No,' I began. 'I'm not going to prescribe Valium.'

Before I could explain why not, she had stood up. 'All you doctors are the same. You're scum,' she shouted, and kicked her chair. It banged into the wall, dislodged a piece of plaster and toppled over.

I tried to remain calm. 'Please sit down, Kirsty, and let's talk about this—'

She came towards me, teeth clenched, face flushed, swiped some paper on the coffee-table onto the floor, and knocked the table onto its side. 'None of you understand. None of you will help me,' she yelled, as she loomed over me.

She's going to hit me, I thought. My heart was thumping in my chest. She was bending right over so our faces were almost touching – I couldn't stand up without pushing her away.

She stared directly into my eyes as she screamed, 'Why won't you help me?' spraying me with spit. Then, a change came over her face. It was as if she'd suddenly seen herself in a mirror. She unclenched her teeth, stood up straight, picked up her bag and left, slamming the door behind her. I didn't move. I sat there, trying to compose myself, aware that my hands were shaking.

The door opened and I swung round, thinking she'd come back. 'Another happy customer?' asked Amy, raising an eyebrow. 'I heard Kirsty shouting and thought you might need a hand. Looks like you sorted it.' She smiled as she picked up the chair and table. I wanted to tell her I hadn't sorted it at all – I hadn't known what to do.

Sister Stein appeared. 'I could hear that little madam shouting again. Has she gone? Someone needs to speak to her and give her a warning. Her behaviour is not acceptable. She's always doing this.'

Amy left the room and Sister Stein began to follow her, but I called her back.

'Yes?' she said.

I didn't know what to say. 'She really scared me' was all that came out and I immediately regretted it. How wet-behind-the-ears had that sounded? 'I thought she was going to hit me,' I said, trying to justify myself. I could feel myself blushing. This was more embarrassing than that time at school when I'd wet myself because Anthony Stroud had jumped out of the PE cupboard at me. At least then I'd the excuse that I was only five years old. And of all the people to whom I could have confessed being scared, why – oh, why – had I picked Sister Stein? It was like asking for sympathy from Genghis Khan.

She closed the door behind her. Don't laugh at me – please, don't laugh, I thought. And she didn't. Instead she sat down and leaned forward. I waited for words of wisdom. 'You're doing OK. It's not an easy job and the people are not easy to work with. Everyone gets scared working here sometimes. But you're doing OK.' Short and to the point. Just like Sister Stein. She got up and walked out of the door.

That hadn't been quite what I was looking for – no offers to sit with me when I saw patients, no tea or sympathy. But as I stood outside and smoked a cigarette, I realised that it was exactly what I needed (the talk from Sister Stein, that was, not the cigarette, although I do confess that I needed that too). I had to learn to deal with situations like that on my own, but I was doing OK.

'Hi, Doctor Max,' I heard someone say. I looked up. It was Tammy. 'I've come to get my methadone,' she said, as she kicked a stone.

'How's the dose? Are you getting any withdrawal symptoms?' I asked, stubbing out the cigarette.

'Nah, I'm OK,' she replied, and followed me in.

I wrote up some notes in my office, and the phone rang. It was Tony, downstairs in Reception. 'I've just tested Tammy's urine sample and I've got the results. You'll have to see her,' he said.

'Really? Why?' I asked, surprised. 'What's she been taking?'

'More like what hasn't she been taking.'

I hung up and went downstairs to the office.

Tony was sitting at the reception desk, waving the test results. 'Red rag to a bull,' he said, 'except it's not a red rag and you're not a bull.'

I took the piece of paper. Her urine sample showed she had been using not only heroin but crack and Valium too. I sighed. I'd thought she'd been doing so well over the past few weeks. Now we were back to square one.

I walked into the waiting room and beckoned her. She saw the piece of paper in my hand. 'Oh,' she said.

'Yes, "oh",' I replied.

We went through to the interview room and sat down opposite each other in silence. 'I'm sorry,' she began. 'I was doing really well and then last week I met a friend who used to be my dealer, and he invited me round to his flat and we started drinking and the next thing I knew . . .' she trailed off. 'I haven't used anything since. It was just that once, I swear.' There was no way of knowing if she was telling the truth or not: the test could only detect the presence of a substance, not how much had been taken. 'Please, you've got to believe me. I want to get better, really I do! I can't live like this any more.'

The world of hard-core drug addiction is dark, seedy and hidden. It gave up its secrets slowly in the confines of my consulting room, but the general public have only a hazy awareness of what that world is really like; how these people long to be free of their addiction, hate themselves for what they do every day, and their bleak despair. As I sat and watched Tammy sob, it occurred to me that for many young people most of the media coverage of crack and heroin they encounter is linked to pop stars. Amy Winehouse, Pete Doherty: this is the drug use they know – glamorous parties, awards, respect, kudos, fame. While countless teenagers follow these stories, I wonder how many also read the reports linking drug addiction to prostitution, crime, ill-health and violence. The UK has the highest rate of drug-linked deaths in Europe. Whatever you think about Amy and the press coverage she gets, she's an icon for a generation. They dance to her music, follow her life, copy her hair and clothes. I wanted to show Amy's fans the patients sitting in my waiting room. They were the people who warranted our attention, who provided salutary, edifying lessons on the risks of drug-taking, who didn't have millions of pounds in the bank so funded their habits through prostitution, mugging, burglary, drug-dealing. For many the cycle of drug use is so integral to their lives that they can see no way out, however much they want to escape. There was little I could do to lift them out of the quagmire and set them on a different path. I could try, but until they lifted themselves, they would always fall back. That's the reality of heroin and crack. No paparazzi, no awards, no million-pound record deals. No life.

I met Flora for lunch again. Although she was working principally in anaesthetics her current job was covering the labour ward and she was enjoying seeing babies being born so much that she had applied for a transfer to Obstetrics. Usually her excitement was infectious, but after my morning with Tammy, I was immune to it.

Back at the drug-dependency unit I had my afternoon clinic. It was fully booked, but as usual, for the first hour, nobody turned up. I sat in the office being 'entertained' by Bruce. He had just finished performing in a four-day run of *The Cherry Orchard* in his local scout hut; a typing error on the posters had billed it as *The Cheery Orchard.* This, I thought, was a great improvement on Chekhov's original and suggested a family sitting round thinking that, actually, things weren't so bad, after all.

Bruce was mortified, though. 'It was a shambles, really, from start to finish,' made worse because the stage had been used the weekend before by the Beavers to get their kite-making badge. Apparently most of the props had either been used to make a kite or had somehow become stuck to one. His wife had been in charge of set design and had collected twigs to represent the trees, only to find that they had provided the perfect frames for kites. 'They stripped the orchard bare,' he said sadly.

While Bruce had had the minor role of Firs, the footman, he had insisted on practising his lines on us. Now with the production over, he insisted on reliving each line, how he had delivered it and the audience's response. 'Many people think that Firs is a minor role, but in many ways he is vital to the whole plot structure. He's the pivot for the other characters,' he said, throwing back his head. 'I'm in character now.' He cleared his throat: '"I've lived a long life,"' he began. I continued to read *Heat* magazine. ' "They were marrying me off before your papa even arrived in the world", and then I laughed. Ha-ha-ha: Chekhov had originally intended it to be a comedy, not a tragedy.'

I looked out into the waiting room. There was Sister Stein's patient, Mr Papworth. Maybe, I thought, he'll have some drugs I can take to numb the pain of listening to this. At that point, two more patients arrived. Just like buses, I thought; none for an hour, then two come at once.

'Fergal, to see the doctor,' said one.

'I've got an appointment too,' said the other. I looked at the diary. Only one patient was booked in: Fergal Anthony. I was confused. 'Hang on, are you Fergal Anthony?' I asked.

'No, he's Anthony,' said the first.

'So you're Fergal Anthony?' I asked, looking at the second.

'No, he's Fergal,' he replied.

Clearly we'd left *The Cherry Orchard* and gone straight into a music-hall farce. 'Right, hold on. What's your name?' I said, pointing to the first man.

'Fergal,' he replied.

'And what's yours?' I said, pointing to the second. 'Anthony.'

'So there's no Fergal Anthony?' I asked, for clarification.

'Yes,' said Anthony, pointing to Fergal. 'He's Fergal.'

'I know that now. I mean, there's no Fergal Anthony, not there's no Fergal, Anthony.'

They both stared at me.

'But most people call me Tony,' added Anthony.

I ignored this. 'OK, let me find your referral letters and I'll try to fit you both in.'

Sure enough, in the cabinet there were two files, one for Fergal, one for Anthony. Both had been referred by the courts after being charged with possession of heroin. Rather than handing down custodial sentences, the judge had ordered them to see me as their punishment. This, I thought, was a little insulting. Since when had spending time in my company been a punishment? The idea was that they needed treatment, rather than being locked up.

My heart sank. I already knew what would happen: I would spend an hour assessing them and start them on methadone. They would take one dose, and melt back into the streets, vanish off the radar.

Fergal and Anthony had been sleeping in a disused shed on an allotment for the past year. Fergal had been homeless for longer. He used to be a waiter but had begun drinking heavily after his mother had died. He had been fired from the restaurant where he worked after repeatedly turning up late and, with no income, had quickly fallen behind with his rent. He was evicted and started going to local parks during the day to drink and slept on friends' floors. The friends had soon got tired of him, and increasingly he had found himself having to sleep outside. One day, sitting with a group of fellow alcoholics and worrying about where he was going to sleep that night, someone had offered him something to smoke. He had accepted, and for the next half an hour nothing had seemed to matter. It was heroin. After a few weeks of smoking it every day he was not only addicted but had also started injecting it. 'I'm not stupid. I know injecting drugs is a mug's game, but it's a better hit, it lasts longer and it works out cheaper. It just seemed the sensible thing to do at the time,' he said, as we sat together in the interview room. Most people, I had learnt, started like this – they smoked it until the addiction took hold and when they needed more in their system, they progressed to injecting. It was certainly easier and cheaper for him to get wasted on heroin every day than alcohol.

Both he and Anthony were injecting two bags a day and occasionally using crack. Neither had been in treatment for their addiction before, and both seemed rather indifferent to the idea. 'The courts said we had to come, so we did,' said Fergal, shrugging.

He had met Anthony a year ago, while sitting on a park bench, and they had struck up a friendship. Life on the streets is harsh and brutal. There is no honour among thieves – or drug addicts – and allegiances formed are fragile and transient, existing only as long as they serve the interest of the individuals. But Fergal and Anthony were different: they were like brothers. They were inseparable, looking after and protecting each other, sharing their food and money. They funded their addiction by stealing, mainly copper wiring but also tools and sheet-metal, from building sites and selling it to scrap merchants. Although they operated outside the law, they had their own strict moral code:

71

no burglary from people's homes, no mugging and no begging. They reasoned that stealing from businesses was OK because they were wasteful and had insurance. While I couldn't condone this, it was a change from the usual ways my patients made money. In a climate where the only currency given any importance was drugs, it was heartening to see two people place value on their friendship.

But that didn't detract from the fact that they had not attended under their own volition and, to date, no one who had come to the clinic under a court order had returned.

I called Anthony in and went through the paperwork with him, while Fergal sat in the waiting room. 'You could see your arrest as an opportunity,' I started wearily. 'You could use it as a positive thing, to change your life.'

Anthony looked at me. 'Can you sign this to say we turned up?' he asked, handing me a form from the police station. I thought of Kirsty and the patterns of human behaviour I was learning to predict. I knew the pair would never return, but I had to go through the motions, give them the benefit of the doubt. I signed the form, prescribed them the starting dose of methadone and they left.

And while Kirsty never returned after her outburst, to my great surprise, Fergal and Anthony did. Perhaps there was hope, after all.

Chapter 5

'And over here is where I was born,' said Barry, as
he walked ahead of me. I was out of breath, having
difficulty keeping up, and wondered why on earth a
maternity unit would be located down an alleyway
behind a railway siding. I caught up with Barry and
turned to where he was pointing. 'Just down there,' he
said.

'Where?' I asked, confused. There was no maternity
ward down the alley. 'There,' he said, waving ahead to
a door and some bins standing in a puddle.

'What? You were born *there*?'

Barry looked a little surprised. 'Yeah,' he said
defensively. 'I was.'

This, I thought, explained everything. It was
clear that he had just shown me something of great
importance to him. He had allowed me into his
private world, and I should have spoken of it with the
reverence he had afforded it: this was the place where
he had been born. Instead, all I said was, 'It can't have
been very hygienic.'

Barry ignored me, deep in thought.

I looked at him uncomfortably, then back at his

birthplace. One of us was going to have to state the obvious. 'It's, erm . . .' Barry looked at me, expectantly '. . . some bins,' I said.

This clearly wasn't the response he was hoping for, but to me, it was just a group of large steel bins. To Barry, though, it was far more than that. I could think of better places to give birth to a child – like a sterile maternity ward. Before I could ask any questions, though, he had set off again.

I was getting increasingly annoyed that a man who hadn't worn shoes for ten years could outwalk me. I broke into a canter to keep up. 'Don't your feet hurt?' I called, as he strode ahead. 'I mean, isn't it uncomfortable not wearing shoes?'

Barry turned, sighing. I regularly got the impression that he viewed me rather as a mother would an inquisitive child she'd been lumbered with after the babysitter had cancelled. 'No,' he said. 'It hurts more when I wear shoes. It feels constricting.' He tugged at his beard. This, I had learnt over the past few weeks, signalled that the conversation was over.

'But surely you must tread on bits of broken glass or cigarette butts,' I persevered. I couldn't accept that bare feet were preferable to a nice pair of sensible shoes. Civilisation was built on the basis of a nice pair of sensible shoes. Where would the Romans have been without their sandals? 'Where are we going now?' I asked.

'You said I could take you wherever I wanted to go,' replied Barry. I nodded. 'Well, we're going to my favourite place. It's just round the corner.' I didn't hold out much hope for this and, sure enough, I was soon wishing I'd insisted we'd gone to a gallery and then McDonald's.

Eventually he pointed down another alley. 'Here,' he said proudly.

My heart sank. Yet more bins. 'These,' began Barry, as he walked towards them, 'are considered the best.' By whom? Is there a government league table of bins? A *Which?* bins guide? This, I decided, as Barry climbed into the first, was turning out to be the worst day of my job so far.

'I don't think you should be doing this,' I said. 'I'm sure we're not allowed to climb into the bins.' I looked round furtively. 'What about a nice gallery?' I ventured. 'There's a Titian exhibition on.'

Barry ignored me.

A security camera was mounted on the wall opposite, pointing straight at us. I smiled nervously at it, gave a little wave and a shrug. 'Hold this,' said Barry, as he handed me a black plastic bag. It was leaking something brown and rancid. He seemed untroubled by this, but I was horrified – it was dripping onto my shoes. Perhaps it would have been better to go barefoot after all. I wondered what Ruby and Flora were doing. I'd bet good money they weren't riffling through industrial-size bins.

'Look!' exclaimed Barry, as he lifted out another bag and produced from it an assortment of clothes. He draped some on the side of the bin. 'Take your pick,' he said, smiling encouragingly. I glanced again at the security camera. 'They'll fit you, I reckon.' He pulled a stuffed toy out of another bag.

I picked up a shirt. The collar was slightly worn but

apart from that it was fine. I looked at the label. Prada! Things were looking up. This was an unexpected perk of six years at medical school. I bet Flora and Ruby weren't getting Prada shirts. 'What else is in there?' I asked. 'Any Paul Smith?' It was like Bond Street, only free. And a bit smelly.

My excursion with Barry had been the brainchild of Professor Pierce, the consultant at the Phoenix Project. Barry had been admitted to hospital under section, which he hadn't been too happy about. In fact, he'd been furious. For several days he'd refused to talk to anyone on the ward, and the consultant, Dr Whitfield, had asked us to try to talk him round. That was how I'd found myself wading through bins trying on designer clothes.

Barry had been homeless all his life. Periodically he attracted the attention of the council, or the police, and was referred to the Phoenix Project, who tracked him down and sectioned him to hospital. It was never clear exactly what his admission to hospital would achieve – he had been admitted numerous times and never shown any signs of long-term improvement. He was now in his fifties – no one knew exactly how old he was as there was no formal documentation so, officially, he didn't exist. He and his mother were nomadic, travelling from place to place; she worked in funfairs or begged, and he was always at her side.

As he grew older, he had travelled around Europe, sleeping wherever he could, in doorways, on the beach, under bushes or trees, with the odd night in down-at-heel B&Bs, if he had the money, or a squat if he found one. He had had no formal education but his mother had taught him to read from a discarded encyclopedia, which meant he had, quite literally, an encyclopedic knowledge of all things from G to I. It was likely, Professor Pierce felt, that his mother had had schizophrenia, which Barry had inherited. His type of schizophrenia manifested itself in a different way from Mr Allsop's.

The symptoms of the condition fall into two distinct and different groups. The first, termed the 'positive' symptoms, refer to the presence of delusions, hallucinations and strange, chaotic thinking patterns. The second, the 'negative' symptoms, refer to a loss or absence of normal traits, typically a blunt, detached emotional response to the world, a lack of motivation or engagement with the world, and disorganised behaviour.

Of course, the terms 'positive' and 'negative' are misleading because both sets of symptoms are negative in that they impede the sufferer's ability to function. Those with a preponderance of positive symptoms, like Mr Allsop, are referred to as having 'paranoid' schizophrenia, while those with predominantly negative symptoms have 'hebephrenic' or 'simple' schizophrenia. This was what Barry had. While it might seem reassuring to have a nice, easily defined classificatory system in which to place otherwise baffling, incomprehensible symptoms, it is relatively meaningless to the patient. They are afflicted with a condition that stigmatises and separates them from the rest of society. However, against all the odds, Barry had found a way of life that suited him, although it wasn't 'normal'. He had spent most of his life without medication, moving from place to place so frequently that he was never anywhere long enough for mental-health services to catch up with him.

He had been prescribed medication to treat his schizophrenia, but I suspected he'd never taken it while he was on the streets. After his numerous hospital admissions, he was given places in hostels, but once he was discharged, he soon reverted back to his old ways. His notes were full of letters from anxious landlords and hostel workers expressing dismay that they hadn't seen Barry for weeks – bags of his belongings were waiting for him all over the country. But he always gravitated back to the bins where he was born, like a bedraggled homing pigeon. His mother had come back when, slowed down by emphysema and pneumonia, she could no longer travel, and it was there that she had died, her body found by the bin men. Barry returned frequently to this spot, not out of homage to his mother but because, for him, it represented security. So, it shouldn't have surprised me that when I had offered him the chance to go anywhere he liked on a trip out of the ward he had chosen to come here.

Professor Pierce had told me to use this as an opportunity to build a relationship with Barry, but as I stood knee deep in other people's detritus, I wondered why Barry needed me. What could I offer him that he wasn't able to provide for himself? The truth was that he was giving me more than I was giving him.

This wasn't the first time I had met Barry. He was a respected, formidable figure on the streets. Everyone knew him. His aloof, detached persona – a result of the schizophrenia – lent him an air of grandeur that provoked reverence and deference in other homeless people. That he had only ever known life on the streets brought him a strange respect from those who had known the comfort of modern living. He was a homeless thoroughbred, untainted by telephone bills and council tax, concern about the guttering or next door's cat. He was also invaluable if you needed to find someone. Although he had no real friends that I could identify, everyone knew him and he knew everyone.

While his manner was of unreserved disinterest, he knew when someone needed help and that the Phoenix Project could provide it. However, as soon as he came to our offices to alert us to someone who was causing concern on the street, he himself would be assessed and, more often than not, admitted to hospital. He wasn't always willing to risk this so he would sometimes arrange furtive meetings with Lynne, whom he had known for years and trusted. Lynne would alert Professor Pierce, who would muster the required second-opinion doctor and social workers, then lurk nearby in the hope of getting Barry into hospital. It wasn't intended to be punitive, but this was how Barry interpreted it. For several years he had suffered from physical health problems. He had hepatitis and periodically would turn bright yellow. He also had TB in his spine, which had only been partially treated so he needed an extended course of antibiotics and assessment by a specialist.

Now Barry had been in hospital for more than a month. To start with, he had protested at being admitted but the nursing staff on the ward had given him boiled eggs every morning and he had soon settled down. They were his favourite food and something he was rarely able to indulge in on the streets, given that saucepans and electric hobs were in short supply there. I had been visiting him on the ward but our first few meetings had been embarrassingly unproductive. I had sat there, staring at him, wondering what to talk about, and he had sat there, staring out of the window, probably wondering how long he would have to endure the company of this buffoon.

When I'm trying to establish a relationship with a patient I find soap operas invaluable in providing me with an opening gambit. I'm sure they were invented, along with holidays, to give dentists, doctors and hairdressers something to talk about. But Barry was blissfully unaware of *EastEnders* and *Coronation Street*, and he had never been on holiday – at least, not in the conventional get-sunburnt-eat-too-much-lose-your-flipflops-in-the-sea-and-get-stung-by-a-jellyfish way. But several weeks into his admission he began slowly to open up. He told me about his early life, his mother, her death, and living on the streets. He spoke in absent, distant terms – talking at me, rather than to me. It wasn't so much a conversation but a series of staccato monologues. He never elaborated on what he said, never repeated himself and never asked me anything about myself.

Before he had been admitted this time I had met him while I was out looking for patients with Lynne. She knew where he could usually be found, and would detour to certain bins that she knew he liked or parks where he would sit alone. He had never acknowledged me and I doubted he knew my name. I would stand next to Lynne, like a mute husband at a cocktail party, smiling benignly and nodding. Clearly he had a deep distrust of doctors, and I knew that even my presence at these encounters might jeopardise Lynne's relationship with him. Then one day I was walking down the street with my mum, who was in town to have her hair done. We had been for lunch and were on our way to a matinée. We were strolling down the street, chatting, when I glanced across the road. There was Barry. He had been given a few hours' leave from the ward and was standing there, unaccompanied, away from the hospital where I had been meeting him. He was watching me and, briefly, I felt uncomfortable. It was a Saturday: I wasn't working or on-call.

Medicine has a habit of encroaching on your personal life, and after my draining year as a junior doctor, I had promised myself I would draw a distinction between my personal life and work. It's hard to switch off when you get home, to put everything you've seen behind you when you close your front door. Scenes come back to haunt you, niggling doubts loom in your mind, and patients refuse to blur into the background.

But that day, until I saw Barry, I hadn't thought about work at all. We had to cross the road and Barry watched us. As we approached him I began to panic. Would he shout at me, do something strange or inappropriate in front of my mum? I knew it was unlikely – he had never so much as raised an eyebrow to me before, let alone done anything to warrant concern. But it was disconcerting to see him now, away from the comfortable confines of a professional relationship. My mind ran wild. Should I turn and walk the other way? Cross back over the road? But if I did either of those Barry would realise I was avoiding him, and I didn't want to hurt his feelings. As we drew closer I turned to my mum: 'There's a patient of mine by the traffic-lights,' I said, consciously not looking or gesturing at Barry.

'Oh, that's nice, dear,' she replied.

I still wasn't sure she understood the kind of work I was doing. Her initial anxiety about me working with drug addicts and the homeless had evaporated when I hadn't been murdered in the first week or turned into a crack addict in the second, so she had reverted to wondering whether I was eating enough and wearing a thermal vest. She set great store by the latter: she was convinced that if more people wore thermal vests, there wouldn't be half the problems in society that there were, presumably because everyone would be too hot to move, let alone break into cars or mug old ladies. One of her favourite pastimes was pronouncing authoritatively on who was or wasn't wearing one, especially when they were on television and there was no way to prove her wrong.

As we drew closer Barry and I caught each other's eye, and he looked at the ground. I decided that the best approach was to smile, acknowledge him with a nod and keep walking. Barry remained leaning against the traffic-light. As my mum and I approached, the lights changed and as we reached him, we had to stand and wait. I smiled and nodded at him. To my surprise, he stood upright and held out his hand. I was a little taken aback. 'Hello, Barry,' I said. 'How are you?' He wasn't looking at me: he was staring at my mum. Suddenly I felt irrationally scared, not because I was concerned for her safety but because I didn't want my two worlds to collide. Part of being a doctor is maintaining a level of anonymity and distance. This is not only important for the doctor, but also the patient. It helps the patient to see the doctor purely as a professional: someone to whom they can tell their most intimate secrets, divulge their innermost concerns and worries, and with whom they can undergo examinations and investigations with minimum embarrassment. The doctor is protected too: in my job I encountered unsavoury, unscrupulous characters so a bit of mystery afforded me some protection from them. I was powerless to communicate this to my mum, though. There was a brief pause. Barry continued to stare at her. Should I introduce them? I wondered how she would react to a man with no shoes or socks on and a long, dirty grey beard. Would she recoil? I needn't have worried.

My mum is a teacher and works with children with special needs. She's rarely thrown by anything – other than when my sister got a tattoo and had her belly-button pierced. She approaches everyone with the assumption that they are decent people. Also, teachers seem effortlessly to project an air of compassionate authority. Once when she was walking home late at night someone tried to mug her. By the end of the encounter he was apologising for bothering her and offering to carry her shopping. 'What did you say to him?' I asked, when she phoned me to tell me what had happened.

'Nothing, really. I told him he was frightening me, that I wouldn't stand for it and he should stop being silly and behave,' she replied, 'and he did.' There was no reason why Barry would flummox my mum.

Without a flicker my mum held out her hand. 'Hello, I'm Julia, Max's mum,' she said.

Barry shook it and said, in a hushed monotone, 'My mum died three years ago.'

I held my breath.

My mum continued, unperturbed: 'Oh, I am sorry. That must have come as a dreadful shock. And were you two close?'

Barry nodded, then told her how they had lived on the streets together their whole lives, looking out for each other. My mum listened intently, nodding as he spoke. This was the longest Barry had ever talked about himself in my presence. It occurred to me that he rarely got to tell anyone about his life without them either trying to get him into hospital or recoiling in horror that he'd never lived in a house and had never been to school. He was clearly relishing this opportunity. My mum asked questions, and he didn't tug his beard once.

I couldn't have guessed it at the time, but that day something changed between Barry and me for ever. When I next went to the ward, he was different. He was still aloof and cantankerous, but he didn't seem to mind me being there, and agreed to allow me to take him out of the ward on a trip somewhere of his choosing. Looking back, I'm not sure if it was that my mum listened to him without judging him, or that in his eyes I had become a bit more human: not an innominate doctor, but someone with a mum, as he had been.

The lights changed and we said goodbye. 'Well, he seemed thoroughly nice,' said my mum, as she strode on.

'Did you notice he wasn't wearing any shoes or socks?' I asked.

'Yes, that was a bit odd,' she said, 'but I'm fairly sure he had a thermal vest on.'

Now Barry had unearthed a treasure trove. 'The bin over there's usually the best,' he said, waving at the furthest one. He scrambled out of the bin – I steadied the side, if only to make myself feel useful.

'I can't believe people throw all this stuff away,' I said, gazing at our stash.

In addition to the Prada shirt, Barry had found four unopened Marks & Spencer's shirts, a pair of hardly worn trainers, which someone had tied together with their laces before throwing them away, a leather jacket with a hole in the armpit but otherwise wearable, plus a mountain of biros, A4 folders, books and a lampshade. Bizarrely, there was a trumpet, in its case, with sheet music still rolled up in it. Who throws that sort of thing away? I imagined a parent driven to distraction by their child's choice of instrument: 'Why didn't he take up the recorder, for goodness' sake?'

'I told you they were the best bins,' said Barry as he scaled the last. 'Sometimes there's even a skip here and they put all sorts in it.' Barry had had to wade through a lot of filth before he'd struck gold here, and although, over time, you could have found everything you might ever want or need, it had a long way to go before it beat the Argos catalogue.

The other downside of shopping out of bins was evident when we came to leave. 'How are you going to get this all back?' I asked.

'We'll have to carry it,' said Barry.

'We don't have any bags,' I replied, and for a moment I thought how careless it was of whoever looked after the bins to forget to provide them for the customers.

'We'll use these,' said Barry, emptying the contents of a black plastic bag back into the bin.

My enthusiasm was waning. 'We could just leave it all here, couldn't we?' I suggested tentatively.

Barry ignored me and went about putting his finds into the bag. I wondered what he would do with the trumpet – and the lampshade, for that matter. I was then forced to endure an embarrassing walk back along the main road to the hospital, covered with dirt and carrying bin-bags of what was, technically, rubbish. People stared as we walked past them. I waited for the ground to open and swallow me. It didn't. Barry didn't seem to care.

Before we got to the hospital, Barry insisted we detour. We walked past the station and there, sitting on his makeshift skateboard, was Talcott. He looked at us with his one good eye and smiled a toothy grin. 'All right, lads, how's it going?' he said. Barry handed over the trumpet: 'Can you give this to Angus?'

Talcott took the case and opened it. 'Oh, nice,' he

said, getting out the instrument and holding it up to the light, as though it were a priceless diamond.

I knew Angus. I'd met him a few times at the hostel where Talcott lived. He was in his thirties, tall and wiry. He always came up to say hello, but as soon as he got into conversation he appeared skittish and anxious to go, shifting his weight from one foot to the other, like a schoolboy desperate to go out and play football. He always carried a violin and apparently made a good living from busking.

'I didn't know Angus could play the trumpet as well as the violin,' I said to Talcott.

He laughed. 'You kidding me? He can't play either. He just carries that violin around.'

'I thought he made money busking?' I asked.

'Well, yeah, he does, but he don't actually play the thing. He holds it and people drop money in the case. He sometimes has a go but it drives people away so he just stands there mostly.'

Barry was already walking off. 'A trumpet, though, that's better than a violin, I reckon. It's shiny. People like shiny things, so they'll drop him more money. Besides, if anyone tries to nick his earnings, you can give 'em a good clout with a trumpet. Violin's rubbish for that.' This, of course, made perfect sense. I said goodbye to Talcott and caught up with Barry.

On the other side of the station, by a row of respectable looking houses, there was a neglected building site. It was between a house and an office development, set back slightly from the road, and someone had erected corrugated-iron gates to keep out intruders. This had failed: there was no lock or chain and when Barry pushed the gate it swung open. Three people were sitting on a battered three-piece suite, playing cards on a coffee-table and drinking from cans of beer. If it hadn't been that the plot was open to the elements and there were puddles dotted around, the scene was rather domestic. There was even a rug on the ground, although it was so wet and dirty it was barely distinguishable from the earth it lay on. 'All right, Barry?' they said in unison.

I closed the gate behind me and stepped out from behind Barry into full view. 'Oh, all right, Doc?' said one.

'You wanna sit down?' said another, getting up and bringing over a chair. I knew the men from various hostels in the area. They weren't regular patients but I'd seen them briefly for assorted chest and skin infections.

We walked over and it was so like someone's home that, for a moment, I found myself looking for a mat to wipe my feet. 'Can't stop. Brought you this, though,' said Barry, and handed over the lampshade. I choked back a laugh.

'Ah, thanks, mate,' said one man, and took it. He leant behind the sofa, produced a standard lamp and balanced the shade on it. He positioned it next to the armchair. 'Looks nice, don't it?'

I waited to see if, miraculously, someone would turn it on. Nobody did. 'Erm . . .' I began. They looked up from the card game they had resumed. 'That doesn't actually work, does it?' I asked.

They glanced at each other and laughed. 'No, Doc, course not,' said one, rolling his eyes and nudging his friend. 'What would we plug it into? It looks nice, though, don't it?'

'Oh, that man you was looking for the other day, he's round by the bus shelter,' someone said to Barry.

Barry turned to leave. 'We've got to see one more person,' he said, and charged out of the gate.

'We're not giving away that Prada shirt,' I said defiantly. I'd ruined a pair of shoes that day, and a second-hand Prada would make up for it.

'You've got to help someone,' he replied.

'Look,' I said, exasperated, 'I can't just follow you around for the afternoon. We've had our trip now and I've got to get on with some more work.'

Barry stood still for a moment. 'Someone's sick,' he said.

I saw an opportunity. 'I'll come with you if you promise to see a specialist about your hepatitis and the TB in your spine.'

Barry didn't reply.

Oh, well, it had been worth a try.

'He's over here,' Barry said, and walked off.

Curiosity got the better of me. I capitulated and followed.

We walked towards the bus depot, went round to the back and there, by a flight of stairs, a man lay motionless. Strewn around were what appeared, at first glance, to be bags of rubbish, but on closer inspection were his belongings. 'I saw him the other day. He wouldn't go to the doctor, though,' said Barry.

I was already kneeling to check for a pulse. It was very weak. The man opened his eyes but didn't speak. He appeared to be trying to raise his pullover. I lifted it and underneath found sheets of newspaper stuck to his stomach. I peeled them back – and recoiled. A large, open gash stretched across his abdomen. I had no idea what had caused it, but it was infected and in urgent need of medical attention. I looked at the man's face. He was pale, cold and clammy, clearly going into clinical shock.

I took out my mobile and called an ambulance, which arrived a few minutes later, sirens blaring. They bundled the man into the back and sped off.

Barry didn't say anything, just picked up his bag, with the trainers, jumpers and shirts, and started to walk back to the hospital.

It seemed likely that he had saved the man's life. Little did I know that, in a few months' time, he would save mine too.

Chapter 6

'I remember falling and thinking, This is it, I'm going to die. It might have been easier if I had.' He paused, consumed by the memory. 'When I hit the floor it didn't hurt, but I lay there knowing my back was broken.' Malcolm shifted uncomfortably in his chair. 'It was a year before I could stand up properly, and I still need sticks.' He leant forward and took a sip of water. He couldn't sit in a chair for long periods and struggled to his feet. 'You don't mind, do you?' he said as, with great effort, he made his way to the window. His movements were jerky and robotic, and he winced with each step.

Whenever I saw Malcolm at the drug-dependency unit I had to book him in for a double appointment because of his difficulty with walking and because we had to break regularly, due to his constant pain. Except for our meetings, he rarely left his flat. An ambulance picked him up from it and dropped him off because he couldn't get in and out of cars. 'Sitting is the worst,' he explained, as he looked out through the bars on the window of the interview room. 'Any longer than five or ten minutes and the shooting pains start.' Since the accident when he had fractured his spine, he had been plagued by them. 'It's like being electrocuted, only much worse,' he said. And he should know. Before his accident, Malcolm was an electrician. One day, fifteen years ago, he had been up a ladder fitting a burglar alarm. It was outside his bedroom window and he was in a rush. After he had secured one side, rather than climb down and move the ladder a few feet so he could fix the screws on the other, he had leant across. He had lost his balance and fallen onto the stone paving slabs of his drive below, breaking his back and fracturing his pelvis. 'I used to replay that moment just before I fell in my head. I saved myself – what? – a minute by not going down the ladder and moving it a few feet. What did it cost me? The rest of my life.' The spinal fracture hadn't paralysed him but had left him with significant nerve damage, which had resulted in chronic pain.

After he had spent months in hospital, he went home to find that his life had changed for ever. He couldn't walk upstairs so he and his wife had had to sell their house and move into a bungalow. They had few savings and he was now unable to work. His wife had taken on more work to pay the mortgage, but Malcolm was consumed with anger and guilt. 'I don't blame her for leaving me. I'd have done the same. I was hateful to her. I suppose I wanted her to go – I made her,' he said, as he looked out of the window.

'Why?' I asked, although I already knew the answer. We had often had this conversation.

'Because I couldn't bear the idea that someone loved me when I hated myself so much,' he said, and made his way back to his seat. After the divorce they had sold the bungalow and he had moved into a ground-floor council flat.

He lowered himself gingerly, wincing. 'And how much heroin are you using at the moment?' I asked, aware that time was pressing.

'I've tried to cut down since I last saw you, Doctor. I'm using about a bag a day,' he said.

Malcolm was always very honest about his drug use. He was currently on forty milligrams of methadone a day, prescribed by the clinic, which was obviously not enough because he was still using heroin on top, but he was reluctant to increase the dose. 'What's the point, Doctor? It doesn't work the same as heroin. I don't want to be a junkie any more than you do, but it's the only way I can walk, for Christ's sake.'

When I'd started the job, I'd wondered why people became drug addicts. In Malcolm's case it was clear. After being discharged from hospital, he had had to rely on strong, opiate-based painkillers, including morphine, to control the pain, as well as diazepam to relax and alleviate the muscle spasms. He soon became addicted to the diazepam and when his GP, understandably concerned about his physical dependency, tried to reduce the dose, the muscle spasms became unbearable. After his wife had left him and he had moved, he started buying it from a neighbour. He began taking more and more for the floating sensation it induced; brief periods of respite from the body and mind that tortured him. His pain was still not under control, and he soon realised his neighbour could get him more than diazepam. Pharmacologically, morphine and heroin are the same drug, the only real difference being that morphine is given to you by a doctor and heroin by a drug-dealer. He started self-medicating with heroin. He never injected it, only ever smoked it, but this habit soon spiralled out of control. When he had first come to the clinic eight years ago, he had been using up to five bags of heroin a day on top of the morphine that was being prescribed for him. It was enough to knock out an elephant, but his body had got so used to it that it barely touched him.

But to say that everything was a result of his pain would be an over-simplification. There were countless letters in his notes from pain specialists, neurologists and spinal surgeons, who agreed that the level of analgesia Malcolm needed was disproportionate to the injury he had sustained. It was clear that he was using heroin not just to manage his physical pain but, like so many of the clinic's patients, to anaesthetise himself from the reality of his life. His mobility was poor but sitting in a wheelchair made the pain worse, so he spent most of each day lying restlessly on the sofa. 'The mornings are worst,' he said.

'Because you know you have the whole day in front of you?' I ventured.

'No, because morning TV is shite.' He laughed. It was at times like this that I saw the old Malcolm. He would often tell me how he had been before the fall: quick-witted, the life and soul of the party, surrounded by friends. Except for those brief moments, it was hard to believe it.

Over the time he had spent in and out of treatment,

he had been successfully weaned off the diazepam, but his heroin addiction remained. His difficulty with walking had a knock-on effect with his treatment for opiate addiction: because he was using heroin while on methadone, he should have been coming to the clinic every day for his prescription, but this was totally impractical for him. In the past, this rule had been rigidly enforced. Every day an ambulance would pick him up and bring him to the clinic. But if it was late or delayed or the pain was too much for him to make the journey, he missed the dispensing times and he dropped out of treatment. The local pharmacies, unlike the drug-dealers, wouldn't come to his flat every day to drop off his methadone and he couldn't manage on his own the journey to the nearest pharmacy licensed to dispense it. After much discussion, we had decided that the best course of action was to see Malcolm fortnightly and prescribe him enough methadone to last him until his next appointment. It was far from the perfect solution, and I was petrified that he would overdose on the medication either intentionally or by accident.

As I did at every meeting, I asked him if he felt suicidal: 'Only when Fern Britton's on TV. God, her voice irritates me,' he said, and laughed. Another flash of the old Malcolm.

'I'm serious,' I said sternly.

'Of course I want to kill myself. I think about it every day. But would I do it? No. I'm too much of a coward. I wish I wasn't.'

This was hardly reassuring, but I had little alternative than to give him his next fortnight's prescription.

I stood up and opened the door. Malcolm grimaced and attempted to stand, falling back into the chair several times before he succeeded. He took his sticks, walked slowly through the door and then down the corridor. I followed him and showed him to a seat in the waiting room until the ambulance arrived to take him back home. Sister Stein was coming out of the office and went through the waiting room towards the interview rooms, nodding to patients as she went. I said goodbye to Malcolm and followed her to write up the notes.

'You have been seeing Mr Wall?' she said, as she strode ahead.

'Malcolm? Yes. I've just given him his prescription. He's still using heroin but he's down to smoking one bag a day,' I said.

'Poor man. I worry that one day he will kill himself,' she said, as she went into one of the rooms.

The door swung shut and I stood there, horrified. I pushed it open. 'What? Don't say that!'

'Well, it's true,' replied Sister Stein. 'Every time I see him I am amazed he is still with us,' she said, in her usual matter-of-fact way. 'Look at him. He is in constant pain, he has no life, no family, no wife. What does he have to live for? I have known him for many years. I like him, and it makes me sad to have to talk like this, but it is true. He jokes about it but, deep down, you can tell, it's what he wants.'

I knew she wasn't being cold or callous in what she was saying, but something about the resignation with which she spoke struck me. At the same time, I wondered if she was right, and what point there was in trying to detox him. Let him keep taking heroin and morphine so that he was totally free of pain. What did it matter?

'Let me tell you about pain,' said Sister Stein, pulling up a chair for me as she perched on the desk. Sister Stein and pain went well together. I was glad she didn't have a ruler in her hand. 'In the Second World War there was a man called Beecher,' she began. 'He was an anaesthetist and he treated wounded soldiers. Many had horrific injuries – legs blown off, shrapnel embedded in their bodies and so on.' She paused, as though to allow the image to sink in. 'He noticed something very strange though. More than half of the soldiers reported little or no pain, despite severe wounds, and did not request any analgesia. But in peacetime, almost all his patients requested painkillers for injuries of similar severity.' She leant back.

I blinked. What had this to do with anything?

Sister Stein could see that I was failing to appreciate her anecdote. She tutted. 'For the soldiers, a severe injury was a good thing – it meant they would be discharged from the army and could return home. For civilians, it was a bad thing, a disruption to their life and routine. Beecher realised that it is not necessarily the magnitude of the injury that is important in how a person experiences pain, but the circumstance in which it occurs.'

I nodded slowly.

'I am in no doubt that your Mr Wall experiences severe pain, but his isolation and hopelessness are as much a cause of it as his injury. He might come here for a methadone prescription, but what we give him is hope.'

I thought back to the meeting I had just had with him. Didn't seem very hopeful to me. Sister Stein read my mind. 'I know it might not seem like it, but we offer him the chance that things will be better for him. When he first came here he was using vast amounts of diazepam and opiates. Now he is not. His pain is not better, but the important thing is that it is no worse, even though he is on less medication. He may still kill himself, but we must never give up on him because if we do his pain will get worse and he will be left with no option but to end it.' She emphasised the last two words with a little nod.

'OK,' I said slowly. 'Thanks.'

I walked back through the waiting room – Malcolm had gone – and went into the office while I waited for my next patient to arrive. Bruce was learning lines for his next play, a Pinter, apparently, and looked up but, uncharacteristically, didn't say anything. Practising those pauses, I thought.

I sat down by the reception desk, more confused than ever. I had thought Malcolm was a straightforward case of heroin addiction due to poorly controlled chronic pain. It seemed logical and straightforward. But I was now faced with a complex case involving the interplay between the mind and the body that transcended the disciplines of psychology, pharmacology and neurology.

'Jesus Christ! Cheer up, Doc.' Molly was peering through the glass at me from the waiting room. 'Bloody hell! That the face you welcome your patients with, is it?' she continued. 'It's enough to make anyone wanna shoot up. Where's a smile for me, then?'

I grinned. Who could object to being sworn at by a grandmother?

'I tell ya, that bus driver nearly got my fist in his smacker. Every bleedin' time they see me comin', and just as I get to the doors, they close 'em in my bleedin' face,' she huffed, then nodded to several patients standing behind her.

'Is that why you're late?' I asked, as I looked at the diary and noticed she had been booked in to see Amy an hour ago.

'Nah. I smashed the doors with me trolley before it drove off and he opened them. I had to drop some smack off to someone. That's why I'm late.' I pretended not to hear the last comment.

I phoned Amy. 'Molly's here to see you.'

'She's late,' Amy replied, as though this were somehow my fault.

'She, erm, missed the bus,' I said. Usually when patients arrived more than thirty minutes late they were sent home without being seen. Often they turned up several hours late, if not several days, and given that the clinic was busy it wasn't possible to see them out of their scheduled times. Also, being strict on time-keeping was the only way the clinic could impose some sort of structure on patients' lives, which were otherwise wildly chaotic and out of control. Some responded well to this, combining their appointments with other meetings or shopping trips, while others saw it as punitive and unaccommodating.

It was generally considered that being late for appointments was a sign that a patient was not committed to getting better. But in some cases this rule seemed counter-intuitive. All patients had to see their key-worker on a weekly, fortnightly or monthly basis, depending on how stable they were and how long they had been in treatment. Those who came late or missed their appointments were still given their prescription, and Sister Stein would harangue them for a few minutes in the waiting room about punctuality and make them another appointment for a few days' time. But those who were being seen for the first time to start treatment, or to restart after missing a few days, or for whom part of the condition of getting a prescription was that they had a key-working session, were sent away without anything, told to return the next day when another appointment was available.

This meant that we were sending them away in the full knowledge that they would buy heroin because they would start withdrawing from methadone. 'You're making me take heroin. It's your fault,' they would shriek, as Sister Stein turned them away. It might have been the only way, but it seemed odd to send them from the clinic straight into the clutches of the local heroin dealers.

'No. It is you who are taking heroin. No one is making you. You can go home, sweat it out and come back tomorrow on time for your appointment. Then you will be given your prescription,' she would say. It was rare for anyone to argue with Sister Stein, and invariably they would go off sulking, sometimes returning the next day, sometimes never to be seen again. 'You must learn,' Sister Stein would say, 'when to be gentle and when to be strict and stern.'

While she could be fearsome, she clearly cared
for each and every patient as though they were her
own child and seemed to know when to tread lightly
with someone. I was still trying to acquire the knack.
'Sometimes they need a caring hand placed on their
arm, a thoughtful nod,' Sister Stein would counsel, 'and
other times they need a kick up their backside.' Usually
at this point she would lift her stick up and bring it
down hard on the floor. I'd flinch.

As it was considered unsafe to give patients who
weren't being seen regularly a prescription for a
potentially lethal medication, such as methadone,
the prescriptions of those who routinely missed
appointments were withheld until they saw me. I
was never sure what I was supposed to do with these
patients and felt a little affronted when I heard Amy
or Tony on the phone saying to someone that if they
didn't come to their next key-worker session, they
would have to see me, as if this was a punishment. For
those patients I decided the best course of action was
to adopt my 'stern face', although I suspected I looked
constipated rather than menacing.

Helpfully, Tony explained that the one threat I had at
my disposal was to cancel their weekly or fortnightly
prescription and make them come in for daily
dispensing, which they universally loathed. 'It's a game
of cat-and-mouse,' said Tony, who had a seemingly
inexhaustible array of animal-based clichés to trot out
(pun definitely intended – sorry, I couldn't help myself)
at any given opportunity. 'The wily ones know that,
really, we want them to stay in treatment so we don't
have much leverage. Unless they're violent, we never

kick people out. They can do as many drugs as they want on top, not bother attending appointments, drop in and out of treatment, and there's not much we can do about it. Daily dispensing is about all we've got to threaten them with.' It meant they had to come to the clinic every morning, often when they were actively withdrawing, queue in the dispensary attached to the clinic and be watched taking their methadone by Sister Stein, who would harangue them a little more. It meant that those attending daily were a mixed bag of patients who had just started treatment, those who were still actively using heroin on top of methadone and those who had been naughty. It was like a social event and probably the easiest place to score drugs in the city.

'What about the people on daily dispensing who are still using heroin on top?' I asked Tony. 'What can I threaten them with?'

He shrugged. 'Nothing. And most of them know it. If they really want to use on top, there's not much we can do about it except make it as safe as possible by having them come here to take their methadone instead of at home.' It felt uncomfortable having to bribe, threaten, cajole and persuade my patients into co-operating with their treatment. In the rest of medicine, patients are usually more than happy to follow the doctor's advice, but we were constantly thwarted by their underlying ambivalence towards giving up drugs.

Amy appeared in the waiting room. She shook her head at Molly and handed over the prescription, but gave her a warning about being late. 'You'll be seeing Dr Pemberton if you miss another appointment,' she said.

Molly winked at me. 'Ooh, and if I'm good, do I get to see him twice?' She waved her prescription at me coquettishly and sauntered off.

Amy came into the office and sat down next to me. 'She drives me mad,' she said, spinning round on the chair and gazing up at the ceiling. 'There's loads of prescriptions for you to sign upstairs. You won't forget, will you?'

I sighed. I was always signing prescriptions. Although they were printed out on a computer I had to read and check each one to make sure there were no mistakes. Inevitably there were. I'd have to find the key-worker, get them to log on to the computer and reprint the prescription. Then I'd have to reread it and sign it. Also inevitably, the patient would fail to collect it and it would be shredded.

I wondered what had possessed Amy to do her job. The patients were rude, abusive and disinterested, and she, as a key-worker, had to engage them in treatment. At least all I had to do was see them once to start them on treatment or a few times if there were problems, and frown periodically when they were naughty. 'Do you enjoy your job?' I asked.

She looked at me sideways. 'Is that a trick question?' she said suspiciously.

'No, I just wondered. Do you, well, find it rewarding?'

She paused for a moment. 'Yes,' she said, then after some thought, added, 'It's not rewarding in the conventional sense, of making people better. I used to work as a nurse in cancer care and that was rewarding – making people comfortable, cheering them up, caring for them. It's not like that here. It's rewarding because if there wasn't this place what would happen? It would all be a complete mess. But this place is here and I work here and, thanks to that, things are a little bit less of a mess.'

It wasn't the passionate treatise I had hoped for on why working at a drug-dependency unit was so great. At first glance Amy was the epitome of cool. She wore pale blue eyeliner with pale pink lipstick and had a black 1960s-style bob. She favoured feminine, floral print dresses and had a slight lisp. Yet at weekends she did Viking battle re-enactments and was a bell-ringer for her local church. Decidedly uncool. Most people considered unconventional are unconventional in a conventional way. But Amy was truly unique in her combination of style and interests. This, it seemed, translated into how she drew satisfaction from her job. I was sure it wouldn't suit me, but as I sat by the reception desk and looked out through the reinforced glass at the room full of drug addicts, I was pleased that people like Amy were satisfied with trying to make things a little bit less of a mess.

'You coming for lunch?' she asked.

'Well, I've got a new patient booked in, but I doubt they'll turn up.'

Just as I said that, a figure loomed in front of me. 'I'm here to see doctor,' he said. He had dark glasses on and a black leather jacket. I'm not sure about too cool for school but definitely too cool for us.

'That's me. Do you have an appointment?'

'Yes, my name is José.'

Sure enough, he was my next patient. I wasn't used to them having winkle-pickers and directional hair. 'Take a seat and I'll be right with you,' I said, and turned to find his referral form.

Bruce glared at me while I went through the filing cabinet.

'Everything OK?' I asked, as I picked out José's notes.

Bruce continued to glare at me.

'Is Bruce OK?' I asked Amy, as I returned to the desk and sat down to read through the file.

'God knows,' she replied, rolling her eyes.

José had been referred by his GP because of heroin addiction. Apparently he was a fashion designer from Brazil.

'Did you find that look I just gave you ominous?' asked Bruce, from across the room. 'In my experience it's a fine line between ominous and menacing.' He did another glare to illustrate. 'I was going for ominous. What do you think?'

'Not sure, but if you were going for wanker, you nailed it,' interrupted Meredith, from her desk.

'I shall ignore that,' said Bruce, glaring again but this time genuinely. 'I sometimes wonder how I work here, surrounded by ignoramuses. The subtle, complex art of stagecraft is wasted on you all. I was feeling particularly Pinteresque a moment ago, but now I'm coming out in hives.' He got up and walked out. There was a collective rolling of eyes.

In many ways José was unlike most of my other patients: he not only had a job, but was incredibly successful and quite well-off. He owned his flat, ate out most nights and wore designer clothes. Unlike most, he could afford a drug habit. While my patients had, in one way or another, started using heroin as an escape from their lives, he had started so that he could live more effectively. 'Everyone use coke in fashion. It just the way it is. And I love coke. It fabulous. The best thing ever invented. But I cannot sleep when I taken it. It drove me mad. Then a few years ago someone gave me something to smoke and I fell straight to sleep, no problem.' He smiled. 'It turn out to be heroin.' He pronounced it 'hero-ween', which made it sound rather benign. 'For ages I only use it when I take coke so I get to sleep and into work on time the next day,' he explained, 'but recently I start using it every day, and when I do not, I get very bad stomach ache and feel awful. There is some medicine you can give me to stop this happening?' He sat back in his chair. 'You give me this medicine?'

I looked at the mountain of paperwork I had to complete. 'I've still got a lot more questions to go through,' I said.

He shook his head. 'Not today. I have to go to work. But you give me medicine and I come back to talk another day?'

It was my turn to shake my head. 'It doesn't work like that. There are two types of medicine and I need to decide which one to give you. This assessment takes a long time. It's important.'

José sighed. 'I sulking now,' he said candidly.

'Are you still using cocaine?' I asked.

José looked horrified. 'Of course!' he said. 'I shall never stop using that. I told you, everyone use it. I just need to stop using heroin.'

In this respect, he was like many other patients who used both crack and heroin.

In many ways, crack is the poor man's cocaine. They are chemically very similar, crack being a solid, smokable form of cocaine; the same drug for two very different social echelons. The effect of crack is more intense than that of cocaine, but very short-lived. As both are stimulants, though, users often find themselves trying to take something to 'mellow' them and help them get to sleep: the stimulant properties last long after the buzz from the 'high'. After crack or coke, a mug of Horlicks won't help. Heroin, on the other hand, is a sedative and works wonders. But, unlike Horlicks, it brings with it physical dependency. My patients repeatedly want to stop using heroin, because of the withdrawal symptoms when they can't get it, but are reluctant to stop the crack. José was no different with cocaine.

I tried to explain to José that while we could give him medication to get him off the heroin, he needed to address his cocaine use.

'I keep using coke. You give me medicine to stop wanting heroin.'

It was baffling that he could view some drugs as acceptable and others as not. There was little point in continuing to push my point, so I gave up to return to it another day.

We completed the forms and, because he was only smoking one bag of heroin a day, he seemed an ideal candidate for Subutex. 'But it's only licensed to be given in this clinic so you'll need to come every day to take it in the dispensary.'

He looked at me, puzzled. 'I not come here every day. It not a nice place. I not want to sit with those people.' He pulled a face and gestured towards the waiting room.

'You mean the other patients?' I asked.

'Yes. I not like them.'

I wasn't sure if by this he meant he did not like them or was not like them. Maybe he meant both.

He reminded me of another patient, Janice. She was a middle-aged, middle-class housewife and I had been seeing her for several weeks. She didn't like to talk about her addiction and referred to it as her 'silliness'. For several years she had been taking an increasing number of over-the-counter painkillers. She was now consuming around six packets a day. They contained codeine, a mild opiate. Her local pharmacy had become suspicious because she was buying so many and she had developed an elaborate journey each morning to amass enough to see her through the day. Her husband was a high-flying City lawyer and as soon as he left for work each morning she set out on her mission.

She had realised that if she visited the same pharmacy more than once in a week, they would refuse to sell her the tablets. To overcome this difficulty, she had produced, with the help of the *Yellow Pages*, an itinerary for each day of the week with pharmacies grouped together by location. This meant she didn't have to travel unreasonable distances. She had managed to fit it around her other commitments so that, for example, on a Monday when she volunteered in a charity shop, the pharmacies she had to visit were all nearby; likewise on a Tuesday, when she helped out at Brownies, and Wednesday when she did a painting class. As a piece of organisational planning, it was mind-blowing. 'Sundays used to be tricky, but I combined getting the tablets with the weekly shop – all the supermarkets stock them,' she said. 'It means I can get some great bargains too. I have to visit three supermarkets and they all reduce different things. My husband's over the moon.' Her husband, of course, was blissfully unaware of the extent of her 'silliness'. 'He's hardly ever at home so he doesn't notice. I do have to be careful about the packaging, though. I'm afraid I throw it all into a bin at the park. I know I should recycle it, really.'

I had thought that a brief course of treatment with methadone, reduced over a few weeks, would be enough for Janice. However, when I sat down and worked out exactly how much codeine was in each tablet and the number she took each day, I was horrified to discover that she was taking the equivalent of a bag of heroin each day. 'But I'm not an addict,' she would reiterate, and I often wondered if she was trying to convince me or herself. 'I mean, I can't be an addict,' she had said earnestly, only last week. 'I pay my taxes and listen to Radio 2, for goodness' sake.'

Neither Janice nor José looked like the typical drug addict we see lolling around on street corners, but when all the frippery was stripped away – where they lived, the people they mixed with, their money – there was no difference between them. Their bodies operated on the same physiological principles and responded to opiates in the same way. Biology was the great leveller.

After much discussion José eventually agreed to come in each day for his Subutex. 'But I don't have to speak to the other people, no?' he said.

'No, you don't,' I assured him. I led him out to the waiting room and Sister Stein took him to the dispensary for his first tablet.

Now Fergal and Anthony were waiting for me, my last two patients of the day.

It had been four weeks since they had first come to me, and every time I saw them I was surprised that they were there. I'd been so sure they would drop out, like all the other patients referred to me by the courts. They seemed strangely sheepish today, though. 'Hello,' they said in unison.

'Who's first?' I asked.

Before they could answer, Tony walked over and handed me their urine-test results.

'Don't look at that,' said Fergal.

I frowned. 'It's no use trying to make excuses—'

Anthony interrupted: 'It's not that. We wanted to tell you ourselves, rather than some test telling you,' he said.

'We wanted to apologise,' said Fergal, nervously.

They both seemed repentant, but that didn't change the fact that, after initial glory, they had relapsed. I could have said that they'd let no one down but themselves, but I did feel let down. They'd failed *me* and, as irrational and unfair as it was, I was angry with them.

I shepherded Anthony towards the interview room and Fergal resumed his seat. I remembered what Amy had said: 'A little bit less of a mess'. Anthony sat down in front of me, still apologising, and I wondered where to start.

Chapter 7

There are times in any job when it becomes apparent that it would have been a good idea to read the contract before signing it. This occurred to me at 11 p.m. one Friday night, several months into the job, for the simple reason that I was starting work. Had I bothered to read my contract, I'd have noticed, in addition to my usual nights on-call in hospital, that I would be required to work occasional 'unsocial hours'. I take issue with that phrase: surely 11 p.m. on a Friday night is a very social hour. Most people are out having fun.

Instead I was standing on a street corner in an undesirable part of town trying to look inconspicuous. I was there to find a woman with a plastic bag. Not much to go on, I know. At least I was down an alley, not outside Sainsbury's. There had been reports that one of the prostitutes who worked the area had deteriorating physical- and mental-health problems. Her only identifying feature was that she seemed always to carry a plastic bag. I had been waiting for Lynne to arrive so we could try to locate and assess her, but I appeared to have alerted the police patrolling the area to my presence. It seemed rather likely that I was about to be arrested for loitering.

'And what are you up to, then, son?' said one of the policemen as they approached.

'I'm waiting for a woman with a plastic bag,' I said, then realised that this might be misconstrued. 'It's OK, I'm a doctor,' I added hastily. 'There should be a social worker here any minute.'

The larger policeman raised an eyebrow – not in a Kenneth Williams flared-nostrils-and-pursed-lips fashion but rather in an I've-heard-these-excuses-before-and-now-I'm-going-to-arrest-you way. I glanced down at the ripped jeans and old sweater I'd put on in an attempt to blend in. Not such a clever move as I'd originally thought.

Doctors and the police enjoy a rather complex relationship. Certainly we're grateful for each other's help when dealing with members of the public, and a number of times I'd been glad of a police presence in A&E when a drunken patient had been hurling abuse at me. But while the police are concerned with keeping the peace and enforcing law and order, this is not the priority of a doctor. I'm employed to try to make people better, even if they are criminals or involved in criminal activity. The moment the concerns of the police are allowed to encroach on clinical practice I start to fail my patients. I was aware of who was a prostitute, who was shoplifting to support themselves or their drug habit, who was taking drugs and who was dealing them. The police would have liked this information but, as long as no one's life was being threatened, what our patients told us remained confidential.

This didn't always go down well with the police. Of course, if they had put their minds to it, they could easily have extracted any information they wanted from me without having to employ any Stasi-like techniques – wave a spider at me and I'll confess to anything. But until the government sanctions the police using biological weapons of the arachnid variety, my relationship with them must remain tense but tolerable. And nowhere was this more evident than on the streets on a Friday night where we'd got very different agendas.

Just a few weeks previously I had spent several frustrating hours at the local police station after a patient had been arrested for shoplifting. While in custody Elaina had divulged that she was under the Phoenix Project and they had phoned us saying that if one of us came down to collect her they wouldn't press charges. This task fell to me and, as a fan of *The Bill*, I couldn't think of any other way I'd rather spend my afternoon.

How wrong I was. Most crimes committed by my patients were crimes of necessity: a means of survival or to fund drugs. Elaina was being held in a grim little cell. She had been crying. 'I was just so hungry,' she said.

She lived in a hostel and worked as a prostitute. I knew she used drugs, and Lynne had tried to get her to see me at the drug-dependency unit. The night before she had been robbed of all her earnings and couldn't afford anything to eat. To my way of thinking, she had broken the law but it was an understandable crime. 'You can tell her from us,' said the desk sergeant, 'that if we catch her again we won't be so lenient.'

If it had been left at that we could have parted amicably, but his colleague, under the misapprehension that we were all thinking the same thing, added, 'Waste of space the lot of them. Bloody hookers and smack-heads. I dunno about trying to treat them, I'd bang them all up.'

It is, of course, rightly considered unwise to argue with a man who has a truncheon hanging from his belt, but I couldn't let this go. I'm not sure why, given that I often felt overwhelmingly frustrated when dealing with my patients. Perhaps it was the way he had dismissed a whole cohort of people, or that he had articulated something which, on occasion, I had thought, only to suppress it.

'You can't say that,' I began. From the look on his face I wished I'd remained silent.

'Let me tell you,' he squared up to me, 'that these people aren't going to change. They're no good, and that's why they're in the situation they are.'

His colleague weighed in: 'There's just one small group of people who cause all the trouble. You get rid of the prostitutes and the drugs and there wouldn't be any crime.'

'But just locking people up isn't the answer. You can't lock anyone up indefinitely.'

Both officers shook their heads.

'Simply sending people to prison doesn't work,' I said. 'If there was an easy solution like that, we'd have solved the problem, wouldn't we?'

'Well, if everyone behaved like them society would break down,' the desk sergeant replied. 'They're not playing by the same rules as everyone else and that isn't fair.'

I sympathised to some extent with his argument, but the idea that prison held all the answers was wrong.

'He's right,' said an older police officer, who had been listening, and I looked up in surprise when I realised he meant me. 'We arrest one drug-dealer, they get put away, and what happens? Five minutes later another's taken his place. The doc's got a point. There should be some lateral thinking as to why people are using drugs or living on the streets.'

I had an ally at last.

Just then Elaina was brought through and the conversation came to an abrupt end.

The two younger policemen, despite their views, were courteous to her.

'Come on, let's get out of here,' I said to Elaina.

The older policeman patted me on the back as I left. 'Keep up the good work,' he called after me.

'You too,' I said, with a smile.

We returned to the Phoenix Project and I sat down with Elaina. 'Thanks for that, Doc,' she said.

'If you had no money you should have come here. We can give you the names of places where you can get free food,' I said, concerned.

She looked unimpressed. 'Yeah, thanks.'

'Elaina, if you shoplift again and they catch you, they won't just let you go. You've already got a string of convictions for soliciting,' I said.

She laughed. 'They won't do anything. Anyway, it's the first time they caught me in eight years.'

I stared at her. I had been defending her to those policemen when in fact she was shoplifting regularly and was totally unrepentant. I didn't know how to broach this without sounding parental.

'Don't worry,' she said, seeing the concern on my face, 'I never get caught. The problem is that I spend most of the money I earn on brown and white. If it wasn't for that, I'd be quids in. I make an all right living with prostitution but it ain't gonna last for ever and I should be saving for my old age.'

'How much heroin are you using at the moment?' I jotted it down on a piece of paper. It came to about £35,000 worth a year.

'That's more than I earn before tax,' I said.

'What you mean?' she asked.

'Elaina, do you realise how much money you earn each year from prostitution? I'm guessing you don't pay tax so your income's equivalent to someone on a salary of about fifty grand.'

She clearly didn't understand what I was saying. 'You mean the government takes part of people's salary?' she asked.

'Yes, of course.'

'Why do they do that?'

I closed my mouth in case any passing buses decided to park in it. 'So that they can pay for things like this place, hospitals, the police, everything. You must know about tax?' I said, disbelieving.

'I just thought the government paid for all those things,' she said.

'They do,' I said, 'with the money they get from us in tax.'

This was a revelation for Elaina, who listened in wonderment.

'So, actually, you earn quite a lot of money each year. A consultant doesn't take home much more than that.' She seemed quite pleased by all this and I saw my opportunity: 'Just think of the sort of lifestyle you could have if you didn't take drugs. How much money you'd have. You could move out of the hostel, get your own place.' I could see that this was resonating with her.

'What I really want is a nice car. Some of the girls I work with who don't use, they got really nice ones – BMWs, Mercs. That's what I want,' she said enthusiastically.

It had probably been one of my most successful interventions and I hadn't been banging on about her health, just simple cash-flow. I should have become an accountant.

Back on the streets things weren't looking good for me. The policemen weren't buying my story that I was a doctor, it was cold and I still had to find my elusive patient. The older officer rocked forward on his toes, which made his black shoes creak. He'd definitely been watching too much *Dixon of Dock Green*.

'Really. I work for the outreach team. I'm a doctor. You can ask me anything about medicine. Go on, test me,' I said in desperation.

The older policeman took no notice of this, but the younger one rose to the challenge. 'OK, then,' he said. 'Why don't we sneeze when we're asleep?'

That wasn't quite what I'd had in mind. How the hell should I know? It's not the sort of thing they tell you at medical school. That's the sort of thing people buy *Woman & Home* to find out.

117

'Erm . . .' I began. The younger policeman shook his head: clearly, this proved I was lying and was no more a doctor than he was the tooth fairy. 'Well,' I said, thinking hard, 'how do you know you don't sneeze when you're asleep? I mean, you're asleep, aren't you?' I was quite proud of this answer.

It appeared to impress the younger policeman. 'He's got a point, hasn't he, Patrick?' he said to his colleague, who shook his head disapprovingly. 'If you're asleep, you might sneeze and not know it,' he muttered.

'Why aren't you dressed like a doctor, then, son?' asked the other policeman, taking the lead.

'So I could blend in,' I said.

'Haven't heard that one before,' he said, chuckling. 'So, you dress like a crack-head to fit in with crack-heads. That it?'

It was, actually, but I could see I wasn't getting anywhere.

By now I was looking particularly shifty because I didn't want any of the prostitutes to see me talking to the police in case they felt we were working together. That would ruin any trust I'd built up with them. I put my hand into my pocket to get my wallet and produce some ID, but before I could the first policeman shouted at me to keep my hands where he could see them. I explained what I was doing. 'You keep your hands out of your pockets,' he repeated. 'I think we'd better sort this out down at the station.'

'What?' I squealed. 'What?' I said again, this time so I was audible to humans instead of just passing dogs.

Just when all seemed lost, Lynne arrived. 'See? I

told you I wasn't lying,' I said triumphantly, and stood behind her. She'll protect me from the nasty policeman, I thought.

'Here, Officers,' said Lynne, producing her ID badge. By this time I'd found my own and waved it at them. I resisted the temptation to poke my tongue out.

Just then a call came through on the policeman's radio.

'Apparently a woman's causing a disturbance a few streets down. She's standing in the middle of the street with a plastic bag on her head and we've got to attend,' said the older policeman to the younger one.

Lynne and I looked at each other. 'You reckon she's the lady you're looking for?' one asked.

We nodded: it was the only thing we had to go on.

The older policeman offered us a lift on condition that I had a look at a rash on his elbow. 'Can you put the siren on?' I asked.

'Oh, OK, then,' he replied. And off we sped – *nee-nor nee-nor nee-nor* – Lynne and I clapping with excitement in the back. As I said, a rather complex relationship.

The police weren't the only authority figures with whom our relationship was sometimes strained. Decisions made at governmental level had a direct impact on our day-to-day work. Just a few days previously I had spent hours dealing with the fallout from the government's policies on immigration.

It was by pure chance that I'd been in the hostel at the time. I had been downstairs when Warren the Warden had rushed in, upsetting a table of papers as I was interviewing a patient for a housing-referral form. 'You've got to come quick! It's an emergency! He's done it again!'

We ran up the stairs to a bloody scene.

All I could see of him was one hand hanging lifelessly over the side of the bed. It was covered with blood. From where I was standing, his face and body were obscured by the sheets, but I knew who it was because it was not the first time this had happened. Several of the hostel staff were attempting to stem the flow of blood from the gash in his wrist. Large clots had formed over the wound, but the cut was so deep that that wasn't enough to stop the bleeding. He'll need stitches, I decided. I knelt down and asked if he could move his fingers – I wanted to find out if he had severed the tendons of his hand. He pleaded with me to let him die, as he always did. The first time, he had cut so deep the bone had been exposed.

This attempt was the fourth in as many months that Aziz had tried to kill himself. He'd been known to the mental-health team since he was fourteen and had arrived in the country after his mother and two sisters had been shot in front of him. He had fled out of the back of their house and stowed away in a lorry, having prostituted himself in exchange for safe transport and food. In the UK, he had promptly developed the symptoms of post-traumatic stress disorder and depression.

He was now twenty, and after several years' work with psychologists and psychiatrists, he had been getting his life in order. He still suffered flashbacks from what he had seen, still woke up screaming, but it wasn't as bad as it had been. He had enrolled at a college, started training as a chef and had moved into independent council accommodation. As he had been a minor on arrival in the UK, he had been granted asylum, placed with a foster-family and attended mainstream school. But when he had reached the age of eighteen this changed. He had had to reapply for asylum, and was rejected. He appealed, and was rejected again. He was to be sent back to his country, even though it was possible he would be killed when he got there. He decided he would rather die by his own hand in this country because he considered it his real home. Here, people had shown him kindness when he had been at his lowest point, and he didn't understand why he couldn't stay. Neither did I.

It seemed unbelievably cruel that someone who had grown up here could have his future destroyed because he didn't have the right stamp on his passport. In the eyes of the state, though, he was now *persona non grata*. He was evicted from where he was living as he no longer had recourse to public funds. He was denied access to medical treatment while he waited to be deported and he had no money. He wasn't allowed to work or claim benefits. Exactly how he was expected to live until he was bundled onto a plane by immigration officers wasn't clear. Pretending that someone doesn't exist is all very well, but the Phoenix Project couldn't ignore the phone calls saying that a boy had been found unconscious in the park having slit his wrists.

That had been four months ago. Professor Pierce had taken Aziz to hospital and, when he was discharged, had made the executive decision that the boy needed

121

help. 'The government can go and screw themselves if they think we're leaving someone who is mentally ill to kill themselves,' he had said. There had been a cheer at the meeting when he had announced this, not least because no one had ever heard him use anything approaching a swear word (by which we meant 'screw', not 'government'). But the reality of his decision was that the Phoenix Project was now, in effect, operating outside the law. Officially, from the local health authority's perspective, we had never seen Aziz. In reality, we saw him several times a week.

Lynne had convinced Warren to find him a bed in the hostel, but it had been hard since the council would not fund it. Because Aziz did not feature in our monthly statistics for the patients we saw, we received no money for treating him. Instead, each month, Joy would do some creative accounting. On the time sheets, she spread the hours we spent with him to other patients. Professor Pierce wrote private prescriptions for his medication, which he paid for himself. Haley continued with his talking therapy, as she was trained in psychotherapy, and Kevin applied to charities for financial donations so that Aziz could buy food and didn't have to beg.

It is one of the strange things about medicine that, occasionally, the political suddenly becomes very personal. Aziz was from Afghanistan. His asylum was rejected because immigration officials now considered it safe for him to return. He told a very different story however, one that was borne out by the fact that his father and uncle, who fought against the Taliban, had recently been murdered. His cousins had warned him not to return because it was so unsafe. Another uncle was still in hiding. As the media spotlight dimmed on this country, and it slipped from our consciousness, the fighting continued. Away from Whitehall, they are still waiting to be liberated. Aziz continued to languish in this political hinterland, unable to work or contribute to the country he loved and that he had called home. I often wondered how he would fair if he were to be forced to return, with his estuary English accent, his British customs and way of life; the trappings of a country that had once shown him hospitality and now treated him as a nonentity. He continued to make steady progress through psychotherapy with Mary-May but always there was the horrific spectre of being wrenched back to a land he had long forgotten. 'It's like being on death row,' he would say to me when I asked if he had heard anything about being deported. He stayed in this limbo state the entire time I worked at the Phoenix Project. I often think about him even now.

The topic of asylum seekers seems to be one of the last bastions of acceptable intolerance, and clearly the government wants to show that they have it under control. They want their policies to appear tough and uncompromising. I just worry that in our eagerness to show that our foreign policy is working, and we are being tough on our borders and protecting our country's interests, we forget the human suffering involved, and that sometimes it is us who are left with blood on our hands.

'Maybe she's having a stroke,' said Ruby, giggling. As we had all drunk far more than we should have, we found this hilarious. Even Flora, who was now paralysed down one side of her body, managed a lop-sided chuckle. We did a double-take. She really didn't seem right. The laughter died.

'Stop messing around,' said Ruby, as she staggered towards Flora.

'I'm not,' said Flora, barely able to move her mouth.

It was the night after the evening I had spent trying to locate the woman with the plastic bag, and I was determined to make the most of it. Now, as we sobered up, Flora was threatening to ruin it.

After months of trying to organise it, Flora, Ruby and I had finally met up with Lewis, whom we had worked with in our first year. When we started work as doctors it had come as a shock that the architecture of our friendships would be dictated by on-call rotas and we often went weeks without seeing each other socially. No one batted an eyelid when you failed to materialise for their birthday party because a patient had become unwell on the ward, or had to cancel a trip to the cinema because of an on-call, or were unable to go to a wedding because you were working nights. For Flora, Ruby and me, this had less of an impact on our friendship because we lived in the same flat. It was harder to keep up with those you didn't either work or live with.

It was now seven months since we'd finished that junior-doctor year. The nurses on the wards with whom we'd exchanged numbers on the last day had faded to a distant memory. Even though we'd been convinced that we'd always keep in touch, it hadn't turned out that way. It wasn't deliberate and I know that we'd meant it at the time – those people had held our hands after we had held the hand of a dying patient, and had taught us the practicalities of being a doctor, rather than just the theory. They had protected us from irate consultants, shielded us from angry patients and made us tea late at night when we flagged and all seemed lost.

I remember thinking on my last day what a profound impact the people I had worked with had had on me and how, because of this, I would never lose touch with them. But while I had begun to understand what it was like to work as a doctor, none of us had appreciated the impact our chosen profession would continue to have on us. The nature of medicine is that, for years after graduation, as you start to specialise, you are nomadic, moving hospital every six months or each year as you build up the experience and skills you need to become a consultant. We were like *The Littlest Hobo*, although no one ever tried to punch him when he was trying to help them.

It was liberating in a way, with constant challenges and change, but also rather frustrating: just as you settled down, it was P45 time and off you went. So, keeping in touch with people took considerable effort that, after working for hours on-call, you weren't always inclined to make. But Lewis was worth it. While we had not known him particularly well at medical school, that first year had shown him to be a quality person and I had felt privileged to work alongside him. Since then, he, like the rest of us, had been busy. He was training to be a GP: he had just completed his statutory six months' training in obstetrics and gynaecology and moved on to a busy job in paediatrics. He had moved in with Dr Palache – or Mark, as we were now supposed to call him – the consultant radiologist from the hospital where we had done our first year. He had seemed formidable at first but had ended up counselling us as we smoked round the bins at the back of A&E. He still worked in our old hospital and through him, via Lewis, we had spent the evening catching up on our old nemeses.

Housewives' Favourite, Ruby's lecherous consultant surgeon – now single having split from his wife after Ruby had told her of his philandering ways – was still playing Casanova and dating a nurse. And a physiotherapist. And a ward clerk. Mr Butterworth, my old consultant, had still not improved his communication skills but had been spotted at the ballet with his secretary, Trudy. It was not known if she had offered him a slice of her Battenberg afterwards. Sad Sack, the registrar, was about to become a consultant, and Daniel, the senior house officer when we'd worked there, had left medicine and was working for a pharmaceutical company. Maxine, the radiology secretary, who was a dab hand at finding X-rays that had been lost down the back of radiators, had initially struggled with the change-over to electronic X-rays, but was now embracing the technological age and doing an archaeology course in the evenings. Life in that hospital had carried on without us.

At Lewis's suggestion we had met for drinks and then gone clubbing. This was a rare treat, but as the next day was Sunday and none of us had to work, we could let our hair down. It was after we'd all had a few drinks and the music was thumping that Flora had made the suggestion that would, ultimately, bring the evening to an untimely end. 'Does anyone fancy doing an E?' she asked, while we danced. Neither Ruby nor I had ever done drugs. Flora had smoked cannabis a few times – but that was hardly shocking. It's practically a prerequisite for getting into Parliament now.

Until I began this job, I'd had a moral objection to drug-taking, not because I thought drugs were inherently wrong or dangerous – I smoke and drink, for goodness' sake – but because of the middle-class hypocrisy in buying a product from a criminal underworld, then complaining when that underworld they funded impacted on their lives. I stood by that, but as we danced, I was overcome with curiosity. I spent my days working with people who took drugs and wondered what I was missing out on. Ecstasy wasn't in the same league as heroin or crack, but I wanted to know whether I had never done drugs because I was scared: scared of what might happen, scared I might like it and not be able to stop, scared I'd get in trouble. I didn't like the idea that I might be scared of something. I was rejecting drugs without knowing what I was rejecting. Wasn't it better to make an informed decision? Society was hardly going to crumble about my ears if I popped one pill. I was tempted. In many ways Ecstasy was far safer than alcohol and certainly than cigarettes.

Ruby shrugged. 'I'm having a good time. I don't need one,' she shouted, over the music. I knew Lewis wouldn't as it wasn't really his scene. I shook my head to Flora, and immediately regretted it.

127

Half an hour later, Ruby and I were heading out for a cigarette. She had just made us do tequila shots, as she always did, and I was now feeling the effect. Flora emerged from the toilets. 'We're going out for a cigarette. You coming?' I shouted. She looked a bit funny.

'I don't feel well,' she replied. 'I'm very stiff and I can't move my right side.' Her hands were shaking.

'You can dance in circles,' Ruby laughed. Flora came outside with us and, away from the music, we saw how unwell she looked. She kept complaining of stiffness and that she couldn't move one side of her body.

It was then that Ruby suggested she might be having a stroke.

'Come on,' she said, trying to focus. 'We're doctors, let's think.' This, after enough alcohol to start our own branch of Threshers, proved quite hard.

It was then that I overheard someone else complaining of the same thing. Clearly this was a result of the tablet she'd taken, but MDMA, the chemical compound in Ecstasy, didn't produce one-sided numbness and stiffness.

Flora went to lie down in the paramedic tent. 'We can't leave her,' said Lewis, and we concluded that the night was over.

Flora's bizarre symptoms continued for several hours, even though she was given fluids by the paramedics. Once we had sobered up, they confirmed they had treated several people with exactly the same thing that evening. They suggested it must relate to whatever the drug had been cut with, but couldn't say what. Something was niggling in the back of my mind, though. I'd seen this before but I couldn't think where.

It wasn't until the following morning, nursing a hangover at the kitchen table, that I suddenly remembered. Flora had been describing what are known as 'extra-pyramidal side effects'. This had nothing to do with the ancient Egyptians, and everything to do with anti-psychotic medication. The tablet she had taken might have had Ecstasy in it, but it had been cut with a drug used to treat schizophrenia; the side effects included tremors, slow, difficult movement and rigidity. It was precisely because of this that so many of my patients were reluctant to take their medication – and Flora had swallowed it voluntarily on a night out. I raced upstairs to tell her.

I found her sitting up in bed. 'I feel awful,' she said.

I explained my theory.

'Oh, God, I took stuff that even mad people don't want to take.' I hadn't thought of it like that. 'I'm never doing it again,' she said. 'Never, ever again.' I thought of my patients at the drug-dependency unit. If only things were as simple with them.

Chapter 8

'You aren't going to take my baby away, are you?' asked Rachel, tears welling in her eyes.

I looked down furtively at the report I had written the previous day, which was lying on top of her notes. I didn't know how to reply. 'Erm . . .' I felt sick.

'He's all I've got to live for. I'd kill myself if they took him away,' she sobbed, putting her hand on her pregnant belly.

I slid the report into the notes so that she wouldn't see it and demand to read it. She should hear it from me, not read about it, I thought. I owe that to her. 'Rachel,' I said, 'it's not up to me. It's a decision for Social Services.' This wasn't entirely true but I couldn't bear to be implicated in what Rachel and I knew was inevitable. Even so, I hated myself for being a coward and not coming straight out with it.

'But they ask you, don't they? They ask you what you think?' she asked.

I nodded. We had discussed this at such length for such a long time that I could only delay telling her for a little longer. 'And you know, don't you, Doctor, that I'll look after him? That I'll be a good mother? He's going to have everything he wants. I'm going to love him so much.'

I felt a lump rise in my throat and looked out of the window to compose myself. The truth was, I didn't know that. In fact, from what I'd seen and heard over the past few months, I doubted she'd be able to provide any stability whatsoever for a newborn baby. 'You've told them, haven't you? You've told them I'll be a good mother?' she pleaded.

'Rachel, it's not my job to tell them that,' I began. 'Social Services are very specific about the information they want from me. As part of their decision they have to take into account your drug use.' I looked away briefly. 'I've had to tell them that you're still injecting heroin and smoking crack despite being pregnant and in treatment.'

'But I will stop, I promise,' she said, sobbing.

Rachel was now seven months pregnant and had been saying this for the past five months, ever since she had started coming to the clinic. I looked at her face, which was red and blotchy, wet with tears. She held a damp tissue and picked at it. 'They can't take my baby away. I won't let them. He's mine.'

'Rachel, I'm sorry, I had to tell Social Services the truth,' I said.

'But they ask for your opinion, don't they?'

'Yes,' I was dreading what I was about to say, 'and I said that, in my opinion, with your current level of drug addiction, you aren't able to provide a stable home environment.'

Rachel wept uncontrollably.

I have had to tell people they were going to die, that

someone they loved was dead, but of all the things I'd had to do in medicine, this was one of the worst.

'There's still hope,' I said to Rachel.

She continued to cry and stroke her stomach. 'If you can give us some clean urine samples, I'll write to Social Services again and tell them. They want you to keep the baby, really they do.'

I think both Rachel and I knew it was pointless. She had had so many opportunities, had been warned so many times that this would happen. Still, I needed to give her some hope to hold on to. Perhaps, though, I thought, I was saying that for me, not her. Perhaps I wanted to believe it wouldn't have to end this way.

There was a knock on the door and Sister Stein came in, as we'd planned. She knew the conversation Rachel and I had just had and, without a word, sat down next to Rachel and put an arm round her. After a few moments, she stood up and ushered Rachel out.

When she returned, she said, 'You had no other choice.'

'It's just . . .' I began, but didn't know what to say to her that I hadn't already said. I couldn't believe I was now implicated in a scene so similar to the one I had witnessed as a medical student, which had appalled me.

It had been my fifth year at medical school and I was doing obstetrics. Much of it involved loitering around waiting for someone to give birth, making tea for the expectant mums and eating the nurses' Quality Street. One day, on the ward, I noticed people congregating outside one of the rooms. I figured this must mean that a baby was about to be born and went to the midwife to ask if I could assist. As I got closer, I saw that some of the group were policemen. They were talking in hushed whispers. Puzzled, I went up to the midwife and asked what was going on. 'Nothing. Best you don't get involved in this,' she said.

'Is a baby about to be born? Can I help?' I persisted.

'Not this time,' she said sharply, and went into the room.

A few minutes later she opened the door and stuck her head out. She said nothing, just nodded. I watched as the people entered the room. For a few seconds there was silence, then the most horrific screaming. It was relentless. It continued as the people emerged with a bundle and walked hurriedly away along the corridor.

They had come to take the woman's baby from her. The door swung open as the mother ran out and screamed after her baby. The midwife appeared behind her and pulled her back. I felt a burning sensation in my chest. This can't be right. Whatever she's done wrong, this can't be right, I thought.

I was overwhelmed by the sense that what I had just witnessed was wrong; an excruciating injustice.

The screaming continued for what seemed like hours. I went back to the office and could still hear it echoing down the corridor until eventually it was replaced by the usual hum of monitoring machines. Some time later the midwife came into the office. 'Why?' I asked, unable to articulate more, but she knew what I meant.

'The mother is a heroin addict. That was Social Services,' she replied.

This was barbaric. 'Surely there must be another way,' I began. 'In a civilised society—'

'In a civilised society,' snapped the midwife, 'people don't give birth to babies addicted to heroin.'

134

I had never forgotten the look of pure anguish on the mother's face as she peered after her baby, or the sound of her screams. I had always refused to believe that there wasn't an alternative to a group of officials wrenching a newborn child from its mother's arms. It had haunted me when I'd first started working at the drug-dependency unit and learnt that, as the doctor, I would have responsibility for the pregnant women who attended the clinic.

Gradually I realised why they were always seen by a doctor, instead of another member of staff. First, managing them was particularly difficult because by the time they presented at the clinic, it was not just they who were addicted to drugs but their unborn child. While an adult woman's body is relatively resilient to the effects of heroin, the developing foetus's is not. Using heroin during pregnancy increases the risk of premature birth, stillbirth and restricted growth.

Injecting heroin was particularly hazardous because each bag was of variable strength, depending on what it had been cut with. Even small variations in the concentration of heroin circulating in the mother's blood could prove fatal to the developing baby. For this reason, the absolute priority was to get the woman to stop using heroin and to be stabilised on methadone. The foetus was so fragile that no attempt was made to detox the woman from methadone until after she had given birth.

The second reason for my involvement throughout a pregnancy was the one I hated. Having been alerted to a woman's drug addiction by the hospital antenatal clinic, Social Services had to evaluate her suitability to look after the child when it was born, and would take into account whether or not she continued to use heroin.

At first I couldn't believe that any woman discovering she was pregnant would continue to use something she knew might kill her unborn child. I had assumed that after a midwife had referred her to the drug-dependency unit, she would do anything she could to ensure the well-being of her baby. Certainly each pregnant woman I saw assured me that she would stop using heroin. For many, this was true. They stopped using heroin within days of my starting them on methadone, and I took this as proof that people could change, even if it took something as extreme as pregnancy for them to do so.

Many were horrified to learn that they would have to give birth to babies addicted to methadone and bemoaned the day they had started using drugs. They did their best to turn their lives round, embracing a drug-free future. There were, of course, setbacks. Some would slip up, use heroin and come to the clinic scared and upset. I doubted that all the women I saw would remain drug-free for the rest of their lives – I had seen too many mothers with young children who had fallen back into heroin use once the initial joy and excitement of giving birth had worn off and looking after a new baby had begun to take its toll.

Sister Stein had warned me though that some women would try to convince me they were clean when in fact they continued to use. It was common knowledge on the streets that those who continued to use drugs, especially injecting heroin, risked not only losing their baby through miscarriage but also to Social Services.

Rachel had seemed to be doing well. After I'd seen her for six weeks, I looked back at her urine tests and was thrilled to see that every one had been negative. I had gone into the office and, seeing Sister Stein, told her the good news. She smiled at me. 'Good job, well done,' she said. 'That baby will thank you when it grows up.' I smiled back, proud that I had managed to achieve something amid the constant failures.

A few days later, she came into my office upstairs. 'There's something not right about Rachel,' she had said, tracing the pattern in the carpet with the tip of her walking-stick.

'What do you mean?' I asked, surprised that our model patient could be cause for concern.

'I saw her yesterday as I left to get lunch. She was standing with my Mr Papworth.'

'She can talk to him if she wants. Where's the crime in that?'

'No,' said Sister Stein, slowly. 'I got a strange feeling from her. She was up to no good, I tell you.'

'Look,' I said, 'every single one of her urine tests has come back negative for crack and heroin. She's knocked it on the head. And you can tell when you talk to her – she's full of how she's turned her life round. She really wants this baby.'

I was rather irritated that this appeared not to convince Sister Stein. 'I've taken the urine samples myself,' I added, as further proof. 'She's not using. Now, I've got to sign the rest of these prescriptions before the afternoon clinic,' I concluded, signalling the end of our conversation.

Sister Stein turned to leave, then said, 'Even so,

would you mind if I sat in with you when you see her next week?'

'Be my guest,' I replied without looking up.

The following week Sister Stein and I sat in the interview room, waiting for Rachel to return from the toilet with her sample. I busied myself with writing in the notes. Rachel came in and put the sample on the coffee-table. I reached forward to take it to the room where the testing strips were, but before I could, Sister Stein had picked it up. She held it for a moment, then glanced up at Rachel. Rachel returned her look, and in that brief exchange I knew she had been lying to me. Before I had a chance to ask what was happening, Sister Stein spoke two simple words, which explained everything: 'It's cold.'

Rachel was flustered but said nothing. Clearly she knew that the game was up. 'You've watered this down,' Sister Stein said, her mouth pinched.

I closed my eyes, not wanting to see Rachel's face now that she had been caught out. How could you have done this to me? I thought, then realised what a selfish response that was. She had deceived me but, more importantly, she had risked the life of her unborn child.

Sister Stein stood up and motioned Rachel to do the same. 'Come on. I want another sample, and this time I'll wait outside the cubicle,' she said.

'But I've just given one. I can't do it again,' protested Rachel.

'I will wait as long as it takes,' was Sister Stein's reply.

Rachel stood up and left the room, followed by Sister Stein.

I couldn't understand how Rachel could do such a thing when she wanted the child. How could someone behave in a way that was at such odds with how they felt? Perhaps she had begun to believe her own lie that she was not using, walling off different parts of herself to avoid the inevitable conflict they produced in her.

Rachel returned to the room and sat down in front of me. Neither of us spoke. Several minutes later Sister Stein returned. She said nothing, just handed me the piece of paper on which she had written the result. As well as heroin Rachel had been using crack, which was particularly toxic to the foetus. Its use in pregnancy had been linked not only to higher rates of miscarriage and prematurity, but also to lasting damage to the foetus's development.

I waited for Sister Stein to start an unrestrained attack on Rachel. Nothing. Instead she reminded Rachel of when her next appointment was, told her she must stop using drugs for the sake of her baby's health, and led her out of the room. I was stunned.

Sister Stein returned. 'Why didn't you lay into her?' I asked. 'I trusted her and she's made me look an absolute fool.'

Sister Stein frowned at me. I was taken aback: it wasn't I who was pregnant and had been using drugs. 'You and your pride are not what's important here,' she said. 'If we are too harsh with Rachel she will not come back. She will go somewhere, keep using drugs and give birth to her baby alone. We will not be able to monitor her, she will not attend her scans, she will not see the midwife and she will not get any methadone. The baby will either be stillborn or will be born alive, not receive any medical attention and certainly die shortly afterwards. We must be careful with her.'

I nodded. I don't want to do this job any more, I thought. I want a nice, uncomplicated job where nurses pinch your bottom and old ladies give you Black Magic. And for the rest of the day I felt unashamedly sorry for myself.

It was Flora who showed me how selfish I was being. That evening, sitting at home, I told her about Rachel and how she had let me down, how no one ever seemed to change, how nothing ever came to any good. I knew that Flora had, from the very beginning, questioned my sanity in taking the job. Of all people, she would administer tea and sympathy.

'We're out of milk,' she said, when I'd finished.

I waited for her to console me. She sat in silence. 'Well?' I asked.

'Well what?' she replied. 'What do you want me to say? Aw, poor Max?'

'Erm, yes,' I replied, 'but as though you mean it. And maybe that you'll go to the garage and get some more milk.' She shook her head.

Why was she being like this? Ruby, I could have understood. She was of the mindset that you just got on with things. She liked things to be grim and harsh, but Flora, well, she was an aesthete. She liked art and flowers and nice things. She bought home furnishings from Laura Ashley for god's sake. Surely she would understand. The one patient I'd thought I was making a difference with had turned out to be a fraud, risking not only her own life but that of her unborn child.

'Look, Max,' Flora said, 'we sit round this table night after night and swap stories. My job's nothing like yours and I love hearing about your crazy homeless and smack-head patients.'

'We're supposed to call them people with substance-misuse issues,' I corrected her.

Flora rolled her eyes. 'Whatever the PC term is, you know what I mean. But of everyone you've told me about, this is the most important. You've got a real opportunity to save someone here,' she said, leaning towards me.

'But Rachel isn't going to stop using heroin.'

'I'm not talking about her. She's an adult, she can take drugs if she wants. But that child has no say in this. He's your patient as much as she is, and you can't let him down because he's totally innocent in all this.' Flora's eyes were fierce and wild. Usually she reserved such passion for floral-print scatter cushions.

It soon became apparent why she felt so vehemently about it. 'You come up to the neo-natal intensive-care ward tomorrow. I'll show you the babies born addicted to heroin. Every time I see them I wish I'd been able to do something to give them a better start in life. That's exactly the chance you've got with this Rachel.' She lit a cigarette.

'But what if Rachel doesn't stop using?' I asked.

'That's the whole point,' replied Flora, exasperated now. 'She shouldn't have a child. You can intervene, write to Social Services, give the baby at least a fighting chance once it's born.'

I got up and went to the garage for some milk.

The next day I met Flora for lunch. 'Where are we going?' I asked, as she began to walk back into the hospital instead of towards the sandwich shop. 'I told you last night. I'm going to show you the neo-natal intensive-care ward.'

I'd much rather have gone to look at baguettes than babies, but Flora was determined so I went with her. It had been a while since I'd been somewhere so clinical. Somehow it was comforting. The unit was reserved for babies who were very unwell and in need of constant medical attention. Many had been born prematurely or had experienced complications during birth. It was eerily silent. Around most of the incubators weary men and women, presumably parents, gazed through the Perspex or gently stroked a baby's face, their hands freakishly giant against the tiny head. Nurses bustled about with trays and miniature bottles of milk.

We came to an incubator. A nurse was standing next to it, adjusting a monitor. 'This is Max,' Flora said to her. 'Remember I mentioned this morning that I might bring him up?'

The nurse looked at me. 'Ah, yes, hello.' She saw me looking at the baby. 'She's lovely, isn't she? Do you want to hold her?'

I hesitated, remembering when I'd once dropped my hamster down the stairs. 'No, thanks. I might drop her.'

Flora had already picked her up. She was adorable. 'Maybe I will after all,' I said. The hamster had bitten me first and, anyway, he'd been fine afterwards. Sort of.

Flora placed the baby in my hands. She weighed almost nothing, and wasn't much bigger than my outstretched palm. 'This is Anna,' said Flora.

I looked closely at her. She was limp and grey. She

wasn't responding. 'Is she . . .' panic was rising in me '. . . is she OK? She's looks . . .' I hesitated '. . . dead.'

The nurse shook her head. 'No, it's OK, don't worry. She's just been given her morphine. Opiate babies aren't very responsive.'

The idea of giving someone so small such noxious medication made me feel ill. 'She started withdrawing a few days after she was born and then began having fits so we had to start her on it,' she continued. I remembered reading about it at medical school: it's called Neo-natal Abstinence Syndrome and is common in babies born to mothers addicted to heroin or taking methadone. This was what Sister Stein had been worried about with Rachel's baby. It came about because opiates cross the placenta, so the developing baby becomes addicted. When it is born, the opiates are no longer supplied by the mother's body so the baby goes into withdrawal. While this is acutely unpleasant for adults, it is life-threatening to a newborn baby.

'Has she been . . . damaged by the drugs?'

Flora shrugged. 'It's too early to tell. Her development might be delayed. The paediatricians will have to follow her up.'

The nurse took Anna from me and I left the ward, horrified and, thanks to Flora, more determined than ever to help Rachel and her unborn baby.

Over the next few weeks Rachel continued to attend her appointments with me. Sometimes Sister Stein would come in, at others it was just the two of us. Whenever she gave a urine sample someone stood outside the cubicle, and Rachel never managed a clean one. She often swore she'd only used heroin and crack once or twice that week, but I wasn't convinced. At the end of each session she would assure me that next week would be different and she would stop using drugs. The results were always the same.

Eventually the letter came from Social Services, asking me to provide information about Rachel's drug use and progress in treatment. In my mind there were two opposing images. The first was of the woman I had seen as a medical student, screaming down the corridor as her baby was carried away. The second was of limp, lifeless Anna on the neo-natal ward. I delayed writing the report until it could wait no longer. I carefully typed out each urine test and the result, then hesitated over the recommendation. 'What should I put?' I asked Sister Stein, who had come into my office with a pile of prescriptions.

'They are not asking for my opinion, they are asking you,' she replied. I despaired. 'But,' she added, after a while, 'if you are asking me what I think, then I should say, do I think she can provide a stable environment for that child? Has she shown that she is responsible?' She shook her head slowly. 'And I might also think, if I stay silent and then the child dies, how will I feel?'

I knew what she would have written. 'Thanks,' I said. She left the room and I stared at the screen. My fingers hovered over the keyboard. 'In my opinion . . .' I began.

After I'd told Rachel that I had written to Social Services and that they now knew she was still using drugs on top of her methadone, Sister Stein saw my next patient for me. She assured me it was because she wanted to help him complete a housing form, but

144

I knew it was a kind gesture to allow me a break to compose myself. Of course, she would never have said this to me. That would have been far too emotional. I went outside for a cigarette.

In many ways Sister Stein reminded me of Ruby: both had a clinical, analytic way of understanding the world that, in the eyes of those who didn't know them, might be misunderstood as aloofness. In fact, it afforded them a unique perspicacity and compassion.

I thought back to the time in our first year as doctors when Ruby and I had tried to resuscitate Mrs Singh after she had gone into cardiac arrest. It had been the first real emergency I had ever had to deal with on my own. I remembered Ruby grabbing my hand and dragging me to the bed where Mrs Singh lay, her family wailing and crying. I remembered pushing down on her chest, breaking her ribs as I tried to pump blood round her body while Ruby searched for a vein in her arm. But what I remembered most, after Mrs Singh had died and we had walked past her family, our heads low, was sitting in the pub with Ruby. I don't think either of us said more than a few words to each other that whole evening, because we didn't need to, but when we walked home she instinctively put her arm round me. I have been at many cardiac arrests since that one and usually feel the need to talk about it afterwards, to tell people how I feel. But not with Ruby: she already knew. And it was the same with Sister Stein: no need for great shows of emotion, grand displays or theatrics – but in seeing that patient, she had told me she understood how I was feeling. I stubbed out my cigarette and went back in to see my next patient.

I was fully booked that afternoon and my first patient was Janice. 'Well, it's been rather tough,' she said. 'To be honest I'm beginning to think my silliness has got rather out of hand. It's very difficult managing without those painkillers.' This was a breakthrough because it told me that she was partially accepting she was a drug addict. She had managed to drastically cut down her use of over-the-counter painkillers but was now experiencing crippling withdrawal symptoms. 'The methadone seems to be holding them at bay until the early hours of the morning but then I'm woken up sweating and with the most awful stomach pains. It feels like someone's ripping my insides out.' I winced. 'I'm having to tell my husband that it's . . .' she lowered her voice to a stage whisper '. . . women's problems. But I think he's getting suspicious.' The pain of her withdrawal symptoms was so severe that she was having to get up and use her emergency stash of tablets until she could have her methadone in the morning. 'I was talking to some of the gentlemen outside in the waiting room and they said I might need my methadone increased. I don't really want to be on a higher dose, though. What do you think?'

Those symptoms meant she wasn't on enough, and although the higher the dose was, the longer it would take to come off methadone altogether, she couldn't go on like this for much longer – she might relapse into using more tablets if we didn't control her symptoms. Eventually I persuaded her to let me increase the dose. 'Why don't you just tell your husband?' I asked, as she was about to leave.

She laughed. 'Oh, you should hear him on the subject

146

of drug addicts. He'd be horrified! He's a lawyer – he'd divorce me in an instant.' It seemed sad that she felt she couldn't share such a huge problem with him. 'I often wish I'd become an alcoholic like all his friends' wives,' she added, with a wry smile.

Unlike Janice, José hadn't experienced any withdrawal symptoms but this hadn't stopped him using drugs. 'I can't do it, Doctor,' he said, throwing his hands into the air. 'It's too difficult.' Because he had been using only one bag of heroin a day and smoking it, rather than injecting, he had been started on Subutex. I had hoped this would mean he could be detoxed quickly and free of opiates in just a few weeks. 'I don't like coming here every day for that pill they give me. It not convent,' he explained, in his broken English.

'Convenient?' I suggested.

'Yes, that too,' he replied, with a shrug. He had missed several doses since he'd been in treatment and his urine tests showed he had been using heroin despite the Subutex. 'I not like it. It not the same as heroin. It not help me sleep after taking coke.'

This was true. Subutex didn't give you the nice, mellow feeling of heroin; it just stopped the withdrawal symptoms. 'Look, we can't keep you on Subutex if you keep using heroin on top.'

He shrugged. 'You give me another tablet, then.' There wasn't one; his only alternative was methadone. 'It mean I not have to come here every day?' he asked.

'No. After a few weeks, once you're stable, we can give you a prescription to take to the chemist.'

This seemed to cheer him up. 'It will take longer for

you to reduce the dose of methadone and stop using it altogether,' I warned.

'I not care. I like the sound of this methadone. It bitter,' he said.

'People do say so,' I agreed. 'They give it to you with a glass of orange juice to take away the taste.'

'No,' replied José. 'I mean bitter. Beerter.'

The penny dropped. 'Oh – better!'

I wondered if José would ever be motivated enough to get off methadone. I suspected I would have to be satisfied with stabilising him on a maintenance dose indefinitely rather than achieving abstinence. He seemed delighted with his new prescription, though, and practically skipped out of the interview room. Another happy customer.

I had one more patient to see: a dose review. I checked in the waiting room and, as he hadn't arrived, I darted outside for another cigarette. 'I'll join you,' said Amy, seeing me head for the door and knowing what I was up to.

As we went outside we were met by Fergal and Anthony coming up the steps. 'Hello, you two,' said Amy.

'Hi, Amy, hi, Dr Max,' they said in unison. 'We've been really good.' They smiled coyly, like children waiting for a reward.

'You've not used?' I asked.

Their smiles broke into a broad beam. 'No! We've not touched anything for weeks. We were going to ask you to reduce our methadone today,' said Anthony.

'What do you think, Doctor?' asked Fergal. They stared at me expectantly.

'Erm, OK. We shouldn't rush things, though. Let's reduce it by five milligrams to start with. Speak to Sister Stein and I'll sign your new prescriptions when I get back.'

Amy and I walked round the back of the building and lit our cigarettes. 'I'm really surprised by those two. Who'd have thought they could stay clean for so long?' said Amy.

'I know. They've still got a long way to go, though,' I said, determined not to get my hopes up.

Back in the clinic, I sat in the main office downstairs while I waited for my next patient. Bruce had recently been flirting with twentieth-century playwrights and his quotes from *Waiting for Godot* had provided an interesting commentary on life in the clinic – not that I'd ever have let him know this. He needed no encouragement. But he was now back in Shakespeare mode. '" 'Tis one thing to be tempted . . . another thing to fall,"' he said to Meredith.

'Look,' she replied, 'will you just pass the bleedin' flapjacks, Bruce? I've told you, I've given up on the diet.'

He picked up the packet sitting on the table by his desk. '*Measure for Measure*, Act Two, scene one,' he said, as he put them down on the desk next to her but just out of reach.

'I'm gonna brain you one of these days,' she said, rolling her eyes.

My next patient was Cormac. He was in his mid-forties and had been a patient at the clinic, along with his wife, for five years. He had been booked in to see me because he and she were still using heroin occasionally. They had been on the same dose of methadone for the past year.

'How often do you use?' I asked.

'Well, it's not every week,' he replied. 'It just depends. It's out of habit, really. We don't need it. When the kids are away for the night, we sit on the sofa and watch TV, have a cuddle, then might smoke a little.'

'Sorry, did you say "the kids"?' I asked. I looked through his notes and saw that they had two children.

'Yeah. Oh, don't worry,' he said, seeing my horror, 'it's OK. They don't know, obviously. And we've got a safe to keep the methadone in so there's no danger.'

I found in the notes an entry from Tony. He had been to their house and checked that everything was in order. But, even so, I was a little taken aback. 'We both need to start thinking about reducing the methadone,' Cormac went on. 'We've been on it long enough and we just want to be a normal family. We know that's not going to happen until we kick the heroin.'

After much discussion we decided to keep him on the same dose of methadone but I recommended he and his wife attend Narcotics Anonymous. He seemed quite pleased with this suggestion. 'If you can stay off the heroin for a month or so, we could think about reducing the methadone gradually,' I suggested. OK, so he and his wife had been in treatment for five years and were still using drugs, but they were normal: they went to work, paid the mortgage. There was hope there, I concluded. They had managed to balance family life with their addiction. I thought about Rachel earlier that day and the report I had discussed with her. 'Can I ask,' I said, as he got up to leave, 'did your wife use drugs when she was pregnant?'

He looked at me. 'What? Course not. She was clean for two years before she had our first little 'un. It was my fault she got back into it. I used to do it in the shed now and then but one day she came out and said she fancied a bit. It started like that.'

I thought for a moment. 'So she never injected?' I asked.

'God, no. We never done that. Always smoked it. Injecting's too dangerous, get abscesses, infections and all sorts. The ones that inject, well, they're lost causes, if you ask me.'

Even in the world of drug abuse there was a moral pecking order. Cormac had sounded rather like those two policemen I'd met with Elaina. I thought of Anthony and Fergal, and suddenly felt defensive of them. They had injected before coming to me yet so far they'd done well.

Months later, after I'd left that job and was working elsewhere, I bumped into Cormac. He and his wife had never gone to Narcotics Anonymous and were still smoking heroin. I told him he should give the meetings a try. He nodded and said he would, just as he had before.

Chapter 9

I thought I was hearing things – and I didn't need a psychiatrist to tell me that this was worrying. 'Sorry, what did you just say?' I asked, rubbing my eyes and groping in the darkness for my watch. I turned on the bedside lamp and squinted in the harsh light. It was 3 a.m. 'You come and see him, no?' said the voice of the Portuguese nurse at the other end of the line.

In a moment of optimism I had gone to bed two hours earlier, hoping that, although I was on-call, I wouldn't be disturbed. This had been asking for trouble. Although my job was based in the community, I was still required to work on-calls, which involved doing a week's stint covering the psychiatric wards in the hospitals and A&E for patients presenting with mental illness.

I swung my legs over the edge of the bed and tried to focus. 'Sorry, you're going to have to repeat what the problem is. I didn't quite understand you. I thought you said that the patient was nuts.' I was trying to keep calm.

'Yes, that right, Doctor. The patient . . . is nuts.'

So I wasn't hearing things. A nurse had just woken

me up to tell me that a patient in a psychiatric hospital was nuts. Between my being half asleep, and her almost impenetrable accent I was happy to believe I had misunderstood the situation. 'Are you trying to tell me he's mentally ill?' I asked.

'Oh, yes, Doctor, he is very much so. You must come and see him, see he is nuts. Two weeks now.'

I knew from past experience that, ultimately, it would be far less painful if I just got up and found out for myself exactly what this was about.

I dragged myself to the front door of the ward and was met by the beaming face of the nurse. She opened the door. 'You doctor, no?' she asked.

I felt obliged to say that I was, although I was wishing I wasn't. The corridor stretched out before me, falling away into darkness. A few lights from patients' rooms spilled out into the corridor, creating ominous shadows on the Victorian cornicing. Everything was very still and quiet, except for the gentle hum of the television, which could be heard in the distance. It's always on in psychiatric wards. If you aren't mad before you arrive, the endless game shows ensure that you soon will be.

'He want you speak with him,' she said, just as John appeared, muttering to himself. In the light coming from the nurses' office, I could see he was young, maybe late twenties. 'Doctor, have you come to see me?' he asked. I explained that I had, and that I wasn't sure what the problem was. Perhaps he could explain.

He seemed lost for words. Again, I asked what was wrong. Then, after a brief hesitation, he pointed at his groin. 'They hurt,' he said. I paused and then suddenly, a moment of clarity.

'Oh!' I said to the nurse, 'you mean his *testicles*.'

She looked at me triumphantly. 'Yes, hees nuts.'

'Yes, yes, *his* nuts,' I said, determined, despite the early hour, that she took this opportunity to improve her pronunciation. I ignored the fact that even though the patient referred to his 'nuts', we should have been calling them testicles.

I took John to his room and tried to find out how long he'd had the problem. His clothes were strewn around the floor and there were empty Coke cans and sweet wrappers everywhere. The wardrobe door was missing and the poster on the wall was torn. Among the clutter on his desk, I noticed a photograph of him and a woman, presumably his mum. They were kneeling with ducks around them, their hands held out offering food, laughing. I picked up the photograph to ask him about it, but John continued to stare at the floor, muttering. I was tempted to tell him to take some paracetamol and talk to the ward doctor in the morning. Then it occurred to me that if he had been on a medical or surgical ward, I'd have done a full examination and history. He was mentally ill, but he deserved the same service.

'Let's have a look, then,' I said, in as matter-of-fact a way as 3 a.m. would allow. He hesitated. He was still talking to himself, but I realised when I looked him in the eyes that he was experiencing a feeling everyone can empathise with: embarrassment. It's easy to forget that someone locked up in a psychiatric hospital can still experience the same feelings and emotions as the rest of us. And there, despite his alien understanding of

155

reality at that moment, was evidence that deep down we're all the same.

'It's all right,' I said. 'It's nothing to be embarrassed about. I'm very used to it.' After suffering quietly for two weeks, he plucked up the courage to show me the problem. It was an infected follicle, nothing serious, so I prescribed some antibiotics and left him. The nurse, still beaming, let me out of the door. As I walked out, I could have sworn she called after me, 'Good nut.'

I turned back. 'Good *night*,' I replied, and went back to bed.

'Why on earth would you want to do that job?' said Tanya, in disbelief, when I explained my current job to her. 'An outreach project? Spending all day hanging out with drug addicts and prostitutes? Are you insane?'

Put like that, it didn't sound like the sort of job you'd actually pick, more something you'd be ordered to do by the courts as punishment. 'Well, your job isn't much better,' I said, laughing.

Tanya was a nurse in A&E. She had called me to help with a patient they thought needed psychiatry. It was 1 a.m. and the smell of cider in the department was almost overpowering. Before I'd started at the Phoenix Project, I had envisaged walking around back alleys, picking up winos and trying to get them into hospital. I needn't have worried about that: judging by the people filling A&E, most of them were there. Several men with beards and dirty clothes were slumped in chairs and a young woman, with two men, was vomiting on the floor. 'Have you got any change for the bus?' someone asked, in my direction.

I scowled. It was only my second night on-call and already I had no patience with those people. The woman who had been sick was screaming at the nursing station: 'Are you gonna clean that up or what? It's a health hazard.' She failed to appreciate that, from the nursing staff's angry looks, the vomit wasn't the most immediate threat to her health.

One of her friends woke up and yelled that they'd been waiting more than an hour to be seen by a doctor, then focused on trying to find his shoe, which, judging from the state of his foot, had been lost some time ago. He burped and the assembled inebriates laughed.

'Great birthday, Clare,' said the shoeless man. She was twenty-six that day, and the men with her were friends from work. Clare wasn't homeless. In fact, none of the drunks in A&E was. I looked on the computer and counted an unbelievable sixteen patients there because of alcohol. I don't mean they were drunk, had fallen over and broken their arm or hit their head and that's why they're in hospital: I mean sixteen people for whom the only reason they were in a cubicle in A&E was because they were drunk. To add insult to injury, most had been picked up by ambulance. They had to have intravenous fluids pushed into them for several hours to sober them up, so there was a three-hour wait in reception because they were occupying the cubicles. The scene was thrown into sharp relief by the plight of the woman in the end cubicle who was having a miscarriage. It's for things like this that the NHS exists, not for people who down fifteen alcopops and pass out. Of course people get drunk, and that's fine. Inevitably sometimes they overdo it and end up in hospital. Fair enough. But these days it happens to so many people that services already at breaking point are stretched even further.

As I stood in A&E, the smell of cider wafted around by an electrical fan, Clare was discharged – and the real problem hit home. 'Just wait till I tell everyone at work on Monday about this,' she said to her friends, as they walked out. They burst out laughing. They weren't ashamed: this was something to brag about. No doubt next week they'd be out doing exactly the same thing. Hopefully I'd be far away from A&E, safely on the streets and working with the homeless.

There have been many theories about mental illness, ranging from the ancient idea that underpins the word 'hysteria' – that the womb can detach and wander round the body, tangling itself in the brain and causing irrational behaviour – to the modern hypothesis that it's a complex biochemical and genetic phenomenon. It's very difficult to prove any of the theories. The brain and how it works, is still mainly uncharted territory, so those who work in mental health are specialising in the outward manifestations of an organ that no one understands. When you're faced with the night shift in A&E, dealing with the acutely mentally ill patients who walk, crawl or are dragged through the door, theory goes out of the window – along with some of the patients, if you don't restrain them quickly enough.

Whatever the true basis of mental illness, my job was to deal with it and get the patient out of the department before they breached the government target of staying no longer than four hours in A&E. The senior members of the team were at home, safely tucked up in bed, and usually things were just about manageable. But I was unlucky with my third night on call. Rationally, I knew it was just one of those things: some nights were busy, others less so, and I just had a bad shift.

'Ready for it, then?' said Tanya, as I came into A&E.

She said this with the kind of smirk that made me feel that everyone else was in on the joke, and that I was implicated in the punch-line. 'What do you mean?' I asked nervously.

'You know what tonight is, don't you?' she asked.

'A night when I sit and watch cable television in the doctors' mess without getting paged?' I suggested, with the optimism of someone putting out deck-chairs on *Titanic*.

'Huh! You'll be lucky. There's a full moon.' Cue dramatic music, wolves howling, and angst-ridden faces.

The irrational fear of working on the night of a full moon harks back to the ancient Greeks. They thought that madness was caused by too much moisture in the brain. As the moon affects the tides, they assumed it must be linked with madness. They should have stuck to writing plays and sculpting. The Romans shared this belief, and our word 'lunatic' comes from the Latin *luna*, meaning 'moon'. Even quite sensible people like St Thomas Aquinas bought into the idea. In fact, until very recently, it was commonly accepted by the medical profession that the phases of the moon exacerbated madness. And, if I'm honest, while I know it's only anecdotal and that research has proved no

159

causative link, everyone who works in A&E knows that when the moon is full the world goes mad, turns up at hospital and the poor junior doctor covering mental health is rushed off his or her feet. I'd like to think I'm above such superstitious nonsense, but obviously not.

'*Nooooo!*' I cried. 'It's not fair.' The nurses chuckled. To make matters worse, I was working a thirteen-hour shift. Unlucky for some.

By 3 a.m. I'd seen eight patients and admitted four, but they were still coming in thick and fast. Just as dawn was breaking, and that full moon beginning to fade, I came to my last patient. She was well known to the department, frequently attending with thoughts of harming herself. 'Hello, Mrs Armstrong. Sorry about the wait,' I said, sitting down wearily. 'It's because of the full moon.'

'I'm surprised at you. Don't tell me you believe that?' she scolded. This made me think.

Perhaps it was ridiculous, but I'd been warned it would be hectic and it had been. Am I sure there's not a grain of truth in it? Perhaps in years to come people will look back at our modern theories of madness and laugh at how silly they seem. I finished my shift, walked out into the sunlight and made my way home, reminding myself that I was a man of science and not at all superstitious. Even so, I was mindful not to let any black cats cross my path – I wouldn't want to work next full moon, would I?

Back for another night of fun and games. 'Do us a favour, Max?' asked Tanya, waving a patient's notes in front of me.

Not on your life, I thought. I'm going to the office to eat a bar of Whole Nut. 'Yes, of course,' I said. It wasn't fair: I'd been looking forward to that chocolate all evening. I'd learnt, however, that it's much better to volunteer for jobs than have them formally given to you. That way everyone is grateful, and the gratitude of the nurses is invaluable if any doctor is going to survive a nightshift in A&E. It's a fine line, though, between trying to help and being taken advantage of.

'It's a bloke who's taken too much heroin,' she explained.

Great. As if I didn't see enough heroin addicts during the day.

She pointed to a bed in the far corner where a man was lying, head lolling, with a drip in his arm. A woman sat beside him. 'Who's that?' I asked.

'Oh, it's his mum. Poor thing. She called the ambulance. She found him unconscious in the back room of her house after he'd been shooting up.'

I went over to the patient. 'Hello, Steve, I'm Max, one of the doctors.' He looked up at me, disinterested – addicts have a tendency to look at anyone who isn't giving them a bag of heroin with disinterest. I quickly ascertained that this wasn't an intentional overdose: he had wanted a bigger hit so had taken more than usual. I told him he needed to be monitored for a few hours so he had to stay in the department. He shrugged. I also explained that I happened to work in the drugs-dependency unit and maybe he'd like an appointment to see about getting clean.

I turned to his mum. 'Let's get a cup of tea,' I suggested, and we went to the waiting area.

As we sat down, I wondered aloud if she had only just discovered that her son was a heroin addict. She looked at me.

'Of course I know. It's all my fault,' she replied. 'I let him do it. I let him inject in my house. He's been doing it for the past four years. I even bought him the bag of heroin,' she said, still crying.

'What?' I said, astounded. I'd thought my mum was being liberal when she'd given me a copy of *Lady Chatterley's Lover* when I was twelve. 'I gave him the money; I always do. If I don't he steals, and then he gets in trouble with the police,' she explained. She went on to tell me that she'd had to take on an extra job to help fund his habit. 'He started using it about five years ago, and I hadn't seen him for a year or so, and then I was out shopping and all of a sudden this man came up to me and tried to snatch my bag. It was him,' she said quietly.

She'd taken him home, cleaned him up and let him stay the night. The next morning, when she caught him injecting in the bedroom, it occurred to her that if she kicked him out, the next time she saw him he might be on a mortuary slab. 'Did I do wrong by letting him stay?' she asked. 'What else could I have done?' When you're faced with a dilemma like that, there's no right or wrong answer. I'd have understood if she'd closed the door in his face. But I could understand, too, why she hadn't. If I was in the same situation I don't know what I'd do.

For a doctor, heroin addicts are tremendously unlovable. They take up your time and they're often abusive. They are part of the flotsam and jetsam that rolls in and out of A&E. We patch them up and send them back out into their world. If I hadn't started working with them that would have been the only contact I had with them. Even in the clinic I found them difficult to engage with. They were like rabid, starving creatures, desperate for their next hit, yet there was a thin, wispy undercurrent, floating like gossamer as they spoke – brief moments when they wanted, were desperate, to change. This was all I had to grasp on to.

Being a drug addict is selfish. It's about the need to anaesthetise yourself to your life, to the exclusion of all else, including other people. Addicts' choices don't only affect their own lives, but their families' as well. It dawned on me that the woman was not upset about her son's overdose, but about the choices she had been forced to make, that she was condoning something she hated, which was destroying her life and her son's. Today was simply the last straw.

'What should I have done, Doctor?' she asked me.

There's a fine line between trying to help and being taken advantage of. But I suppose when you love someone the line gets blurred.

'Why won't anyone help me?' said Mr Jacobs, as he lunged at me. I moved aside and he clattered into a trolley. Tanya and another nurse rolled their eyes and corralled him back into the side room. He began swearing at them, to which they made no response. 'Get me a cup of tea, will you, love?' he said, as Tanya walked out of the door. She didn't turn back.

From outside I could hear someone screaming drunkenly. As I was talking to Mr Jacobs another man wandered into the room, looking for the toilet.

He could barely stand and a casualty officer ordered him back to his cubicle, advising him to avoid the puddle on the floor where Mr Jacobs had just vomited. Welcome to A&E on a Friday evening.

My last night and it couldn't end soon enough. Mr Jacobs was demanding to be seen because he wanted help. He couldn't specify exactly what this help would entail, but it seemed he wanted us to stop him drinking. He was drunk. He had tried alcohol detox programmes but hadn't lasted more than a few weeks before going back to the bottle. He seemed to think that this was the fault of alcohol services, because they wouldn't 'do enough'. The answer to Mr Jacobs' question as to why someone wouldn't help him was that no one could until he started to take responsibility for his drinking. Only one person could stop him drinking, and that person was himself. He could be helped, but he had to make a commitment to remain sober and stick to it.

Alcohol is the most commonly used drug in the UK, and the most commonly abused. In A&E its effects are there for all to see, from the homeless person who uses it to block out the bleak reality of life to the binge-drinking shoeless teenager surrounded by giddy friends texting each other. There are the occasional users who've over-indulged and the hardened alcoholic who drinks from dawn till dusk. There's the thirty-something woman now looking for the morning-after pill, the inebriated businessman who's collapsed and banged his head, louts with bloody noses, and gin-swigging old ladies. In A&E, you'd be forgiven for thinking we were in the throes of a drunkenness epidemic. Of course, that isn't true.

But what A&E teaches you is that nothing changes until people take responsibility for their actions. I've been struck by the amount of resources that those who use alcohol take up as a result of the choices they make. Drug addicts and the homeless rely heavily on services too, but alcohol is by far the major problem. And it's not alcohol that smashes up cars, punches people or throws bricks through windows. It's a person who decided to get drunk and behave like that. Drunken hooligans won't change their ways until responsibility for their behaviour is put squarely at their feet.

Back in A&E, Tanya gave Mr Jacobs a mop and instructed him on how to use it. That sobered him up.

'You're joking, aren't you?' I laughed.

Mrs Green was ashen-faced. 'No, I'm serious.'

The smile slid from my face. I stared at her in disbelief.

Mrs Green was in her fifties. She worked in a local nursing home, had two grown-up children and was married. Last night she had tried to commit suicide. In the cheery world of psychiatry, this was hardly news, but what I found so hard to accept was that, too scared to do the deed herself, she had persuaded someone to do it for her. For twenty pounds someone had injected her with a lethal dose of heroin. Unfortunately – or thankfully – the heroin Mrs Green had bought had been cut with so many other things that its potency had been diluted so far that it didn't kill her. She'd lain in a coma on a street for a few hours before someone had spotted her and called an ambulance. After Flora's experience, I dreaded to think what the unscrupulous drug-dealer had cut the heroin with, but whatever it was, it hadn't appeared to do her much harm and, in a way, I was heartened that someone else's greed could have such a positive effect on another's life.

The thing I couldn't get over was that someone had actually agreed to commit what constituted murder for a mere twenty pounds. Was life really so cheap on the streets, these days?

'I gave him my watch as well – and do you know the annoying thing?' she asked.

'Do tell me,' I said, trying to imagine what could be worse than discovering your life is worth just twenty pounds and an Argos watch.

'When I came round in A&E, he'd pinched my earrings too. I mean, what would he want with those?'

She really hadn't had a good day. She told me that she had tried to kill herself or, rather, paid someone else to botch the job, because that morning she'd received her credit-card bill. 'I'd never be able to pay it all off, I knew that. Then my husband saw it and he blew up at me. I felt like a failure.' Her bills had been mounting over the past few years so that now she owed more than eight times her salary.

Lots of people could be blamed for the situation Mrs Green had got into, not least Mrs Green herself. Credit cards, in a similar way to drugs, work on the idea of instantaneous gratification, and what could be more appealing to someone like Mrs Green? She didn't have much fun in her life. Her husband had MS, they lived in a small council flat, she worked in a poorly paid job. She had run up those huge bills buying things she couldn't afford to try to make herself feel better. In our society, to be someone you must consume. Happiness is available at a store near you – with a price tag, of course.

In the morning, as my night shift was ending, I went to discharge Mrs Green as her blood-test results had come back normal. Her husband and two children were round her bed, telling her how much they loved her and how she mustn't worry. There are some things in life that money – or, indeed, a credit card – really can't buy.

Chapter 10

That night there had been blood everywhere. Unaware at the time of what the other was going through, it wasn't until it was all over and we could compare stories, dazed and shocked at the kitchen table, that Ruby and I saw how we had both, in different ways, been lucky.

That evening we had gone out to meet Lewis and Supriya. Ruby was still working and had promised to meet us later. We had gone out for dinner on the pretext of celebrating Supriya's birthday although it had been so long ago, and we had rearranged so many times, that this was forgotten. Supriya was run off her feet doing a job in oncology – cancer – as part of her training in general medicine. Her aim was to become a consultant physician in a teaching hospital, doing research as well as clinical work. She was particularly interested in the kidneys. None of us could see the appeal: those funny little bean-shaped organs were the cause of constant anguish not only to us as medical students, where their role in just about every bodily function baffled us, but also as doctors, where they had an annoying habit of stopping working in our patients just when we thought things were going well. 'The only time I'm interested in kidneys is when they're combined with steak and put in a pie,' said Lewis.

Supriya huffed. 'They're fascinating. Take their role in the renin-angiotensin system—'

'No!' we chorused.

'First rule of the evening: no kidney discussion,' said Lewis, folding his arms.

'You're a fine one to talk,' said Supriya. 'At least everyone's got kidneys. You're always going on about things no one's even heard of.'

This was true. Although Lewis was currently working in paediatrics, as part of his training to be a GP, he wanted ultimately to work in sports medicine. However, outside this, he had a well-known predilection for eponymous syndromes. These are conditions defined by a constellation of symptoms and named after the doctor who had first described them. As a group of conditions, they were the weirdest and rarest. Knowledge of them was generally of absolutely no use in clinical practice but guaranteed to get you so many Brownie points in exams that you could have set up your own pack. I was sure this was why Lewis had done so well at medical school: he had blinded the examiners with conditions that even they had never heard of.

One of his favourite eponymous syndromes was Leriche's Syndrome – don't worry about how to pronounce it: I can assure you that you'll never need to say it, not even in a game of Trivial Pursuit. It was made up of a triad of symptoms: absence of the pulses in the legs, pain on walking and impotence. Lewis collected medical obscurities as other people collect stamps – which would have been far less irritating. In fact, when I was listening to him go into tedious detail about some rare-as-hen's-teeth condition, I often worried that I had Gélineau's syndrome – a condition affecting young men who are overcome by the irresistible desire to sleep in socially inappropriate situations. Oh, God, he's got me at it now.

'OK, no mention of obscure medical conditions,' agreed Lewis.

'And no mention of babies, either,' I said, looking pointedly at Flora.

'Aw, babies,' said Flora, immediately moist-eyed. 'You should see their little crumpled faces when they come out. You just want to eat them.'

'See what I mean?' I muttered to the others.

Prohibited medical conversations aside, the rest of the evening went well. It was good to catch up with Supriya especially. While the hospital where she now worked was not very far away, we rarely saw her. She was living in hospital accommodation and spent every spare minute – of which she didn't have many – studying for exams. She was determined to scurry up the slippery pole of medical careers as quickly as possible. 'I can't stand being shouted at every time something goes wrong for much longer. I want to be the one doing the shouting,' she said, rubbing her hands. We all nodded.

It seemed that, finally, we were beginning to find areas of medicine that we enjoyed and wanted to work in. Last year, I wouldn't have believed it was possible.

We had all, at different points, experienced difficulty even staying in medicine, let alone finding areas we wanted to specialise in. I realised, with growing dread, that when this year at the Phoenix Project was over and I began my next year of work I, too, would have to study for exams. I'd been sitting them since I was eleven and had at least another four years' worth ahead. Your medical degree was just the start. It merely enabled you to put two letters in front of your name and hold a stethoscope with some authority. The real job of training to be a doctor – a proper doctor, that is, rather than someone who puts their fingers up people's bottoms all day every day or prescribes what others tell them to – had only just begun and involved several post-graduate examinations. Over the next few years, we had to become more than competent: we had to be excellent.

After the meal we went to a bar. The idea had been to get blind drunk but Supriya couldn't resist trying to tell us about the effects of alcohol on the kidney, which took the fun out of it. It also prompted Lewis into spouting an alcohol-related eponymous syndrome characterised by the inability to form new memories due to deficiency in thiamine. (Korsakoff's syndrome, in case you were wondering and, no, you're never going to need to know how to pronounce that one, either.) 'It does seem strange, though,' continued Supriya, looking at me and ignoring Lewis, 'that you spend all day dealing with people addicted to drugs yet here we are smoking and drinking. If they tried to introduce either alcohol or tobacco now, it would be banned, wouldn't it?'

She had a point. 'But if there were no tobacco and alcohol, we'd find something else to replace them,' I said.

'I'm going for a fag,' said Flora.

It was shortly after this that the evening took an unusual turn and I nearly died. Ruby never arrived for the reason that at around the time we were leaving the bar, she was on the other side of town with her hand inside a young man's chest. Not, of course, that we knew this as we left the bar.

Supriya was on-call over the weekend so we saw her into a cab. As it was a Friday night, and Lewis, Flora and I weren't working the next day, we decided to go for a kebab. Well, Lewis decided that; Flora and I are vegetarian. 'We can have lettuce in pitta bread,' said Flora, sneering.

'They do falafels,' said Lewis, helpfully, and off we went.

'What's happened to Ruby? I thought she was supposed to meet us in the bar,' said Flora, as we walked along the pavement.

'I hope she didn't arrive just after we'd gone,' said Lewis.

They walked ahead and I tried to call her. No answer. I'd already texted her twice and she hadn't replied. I looked at my watch. It was now 11.20. She was supposed to finish at 9. Even if she'd been delayed, there was no way she would still be at work at this time, I thought. I passed a bank and went round the side to use the cash machine as I tried to phone her again.

When I turned round three people were standing in front of me. I still had the phone to my ear and absentmindedly stepped aside to let them get to the cash machine.

They moved to block my path. 'You a doctor, yeah?' said one.

I wondered if I knew him. I was sure I didn't. I was rather puzzled as to how he knew my profession. 'Sorry, do I know you?' I asked.

'You will be sorry,' said another, as he moved closer. 'Now, don't play games with us, we know you're a doctor. What drugs you got on you?'

I found the notion that doctors wandered round with pocketfuls of tablets rather funny. 'What?' I said, laughing. 'I haven't got any drugs on me.' I tried to walk back to the main street.

One of the men pushed me against the wall. 'Take him over there and get his money out,' said another to the man who was holding me.

Inexplicably, until now I hadn't been scared, just intrigued as to how they knew I was a doctor. But suddenly it dawned on me that I was about to be mugged. If the men had got me to the cashpoint they would have received a salutary lesson in how doctors, contrary to popular belief, are not paid particularly handsomely for their efforts: my account was significantly overdrawn. But before that could happen someone came round the corner. It was a woman in her early twenties, in a short skirt, boots and a flimsy jacket. She was hugging herself for warmth. Now, she was someone I did recognise. I couldn't put a name to her, though, and racked my brains. To my dismay, however, it was soon clear that she knew the men.

'You said you wouldn't hurt him,' she told the first man.

'Shut up,' he snarled.

She looked at me furtively, but as our eyes met she glanced away. I did know her: she was friends with one of Lynne's patients. I'd seen her a few times in the women's hostel I visited. I still couldn't remember her name but she and Lynne's patient were prostitutes. A moment of clarity: one of these men was probably her pimp; she'd spotted me walking down the road, told them who I was, and they had seen an opportunity. I felt a bit sick and incredibly stupid.

I had naïvely thought I would be immune from the unsavoury characters who inhabited the world in which I worked. Why had I thought I would be protected because I worked with them? If anything, it made me stand out more. Lynne had warned me to be careful and I had dismissed this as scaremongering. I'd been cocky. Since I'd started my job, people I would previously have avoided now waved at me and smiled. Stupidly I had thought this meant I was safe. I knew only a fraction of the people on the streets, and while my patients might not attack me, that didn't mean no one else would.

I didn't know what to do. It was unlikely that I'd be able to reason with the men and it didn't seem the right moment to try to recruit them for treatment at the drug-dependency unit. Alternatively, I couldn't have fought my way out of a catheter bag, let alone fend off three assailants. But I was also damn sure I wasn't going to hand over money I'd earned from trying to help people like them (OK, technically I was overdrawn so it was the bank's money, but that's a moot point).

It was then that Barry appeared. To this day I don't know where he came from but he had obviously seen what was happening and decided to intervene. 'Leave him alone,' he said, walking boldly into the middle of the group. He was much shorter than the others but he stood firm.

'Fuck off, Granddad,' said the first man.

'Leave him alone,' Barry repeated in his monotone.

To my amazement, the man holding me against the wall let me go.

'I know who you are and you'll be sorry,' said Barry, staring at the man who had been doing most of the talking.

The events that followed were over in a matter of seconds. One man pulled a knife. The girl screamed and grabbed him round the neck. He hit her across the face, sending her crashing to the ground, then turned and kicked her. I stepped forward and pushed him off her. He lunged at me. Barry raised his hand and leant forward, then fell into me. The next thing I knew I was covered with blood, the men were gone, and Barry and the girl were lying on the pavement.

I stood there, dazed, for a few seconds, then looked down to see where the blood was coming from. It was on my hands and shirt, but I couldn't find a wound. Suddenly I realised the blood wasn't mine, it was Barry's. I panicked, then slipped into the calm of doctor-mode: he was moving. 'Don't get up,' I said, as I bent over him.

In the scuffle he had hit his head and was still quite dazed. There was a nasty cut on the side of his head, which was bleeding profusely. But that didn't account for the amount on me. I glanced down and saw blood pouring from his arm. He lifted it towards his face, and blood spurted over me and onto the pavement. He must have grabbed the knife, and as the man had pulled away it had sliced through his hand.

The girl got up. 'Go and get help,' I said, and she ran towards the main road.

Just then, Flora and Lewis appeared. 'Oh, my God!' cried Flora. They threw down their kebabs and raced towards me.

'Find the wound,' said Lewis, kneeling to attend to Barry, while Flora tried to rip my shirt off.

Buttons flew in all directions, and I was perplexed until it dawned on me how awful I must look. 'It's not me – I'm not bleeding,' I said. 'It's him. He's been stabbed in the hand.' I pointed at Barry.

Flora visibly relaxed. 'Let me check anyway. You can't always tell,' she said, and ran her ice-cold hands over my body.

Satisfied that I wasn't bleeding, she turned to Barry. It was interesting to see her and Lewis work so effectively together. It was like being back on the ward and, fleetingly, I was proud of how composed and professional they were in an emergency. Lewis had sat Barry against the wall and elevated his hand above his head. 'I need a belt,' he said, and Flora turned to me.

'Great. I lose a shirt and a belt in one evening,' I said, as I took it off and handed it over, pleased that I was managing to joke at such a time.

'Shut up. I've just thrown away an uneaten falafel kebab because of you,' Flora said, as she passed it to Lewis. *Touché.*

The ambulance came and we went with Barry to the hospital. It was the same hospital where Flora worked, which was linked to my drug-dependency unit and where I did on-calls, so everyone fussed around us and treated Barry like royalty when we explained he had saved my life. He had to wait for the hand specialist from the plastic-surgery department to come in but they would admit him for monitoring so we left him and went home.

Lewis came with us. He lived nearer to the hospital than we did, but we were high on adrenalin and knew there was no question that he'd go home until we'd had a cup of tea and debriefed. I'd borrowed surgical scrubs from A&E as my shirt was ruined, and we got a taxi back.

We opened the door to find Ruby sitting at the kitchen table drinking a glass of wine. 'There you are!' I exclaimed.

'There was a stabbing,' interrupted Flora, 'blood everywhere. Max could have died.'

'You all right, Ruby?' said Lewis, sitting down.

'I was involved in a stabbing too,' she replied – and this is where the story of Ruby's night begins.

Ruby had been on-call, working on the orthopaedic ward. There were some acutely unwell patients and she had stayed late to make sure they would be stable over the weekend. Eventually she left the ward and, having had nothing to eat since lunchtime and knowing she had missed dinner with us, stopped off at the vending machine in the A&E reception area for a bar of chocolate and some coffee. 'It'd run out of KitKats. They always run out of KitKats,' she said, diverting from the story. 'I had to get a Lion Bar, and they're just not the same, are they?'

'Get on with the story,' we said, from the edge of our seats.

As she'd walked through A&E, a trauma call went out. 'ETA two minutes. Open chest wound,' a nurse shouted. Ruby had stopped to chat to one of the social workers and watched as the trauma team congregated at the ambulance-bay entrance. It was then she realised there wasn't a trauma surgeon.

The trauma team is made up of a selection of different specialities, including anaesthetists, A&E nurses, doctors and surgeons.

'Where's the surgeon?' she said to the lead nurse. Everyone looked around. At that moment Ruby realised that the on-call surgical registrar was still in theatre doing an emergency operation. 'If it's an open chest wound, you should have a trauma surgeon here. He'll need bilateral chest drains,' she said.

'The surgeon's over there,' said the nurse, pointing to a petrified junior doctor, who was trying to get his latex gloves on.

'He's not a surgeon. He's a junior doctor. Can you do a chest drain?' Ruby shouted to him. He looked at her and shook his head as a boy was rushed in on a stretcher surrounded by police and ambulance crew.

'Quick!' shouted a paramedic, as they raced him through to Re-sus. 'We're losing him.'

'Multiple stab wounds to chest and back,' shouted another paramedic, to the assembled team, as they got to work.

Ruby stood at the entrance for a few moments, hesitating. She took a deep breath, dropped her bag and ran over to help. While the anaesthetist concentrated on his airway, she took a scalpel to insert the first chest drain. 'Come on!' she said, to the junior doctor, who was hiding behind her. 'Watch me do this one and I'll help you with the other.' The boy had been stabbed in the chest, which had caused him to haemorrhage blood into his lungs, a condition known as a haemothorax, making breathing difficult. The drains would draw out the blood and enable oxygen to get into his lungs. 'He's losing output,' said a nurse.

'Get fluids into him – fast!' shouted the anaesthetist.

Suddenly everyone paused. 'He's gone into cardiac arrest,' yelled a nurse. He had lost so much blood that his heart had stopped beating and he was dying. Someone began chest compressions.

'No,' said Ruby, looking at the anaesthetist. 'He's bleeding from somewhere. His heart won't start again unless we find where he's been bleeding.'

'We don't have time to get a cardiothoracic surgeon,' said the anaesthetist.

She turned to the casualty doctor. 'He'll die if we don't do something. He needs a clam-shell thoracotomy,' she said. Several nurses said they didn't even know what that was.

Ruby swallowed hard. 'OK, I'll do it,' she said. 'Get me a saw.' She still had the scalpel in her hand from doing the chest drain so she used it to make an incision across his chest.

'Oh, my God,' said the junior doctor as he watched what was happening.

Ruby lifted the skin and began to cut through the underlying muscle that attaches the ribcage to the breastplate.

A nurse returned, out of breath. 'We can't find a saw,' she said, panicking.

Ruby thought for a moment. 'Get me scissors, then.'

'What?' said the nurse.

'Scissors! Get me scissors,' repeated Ruby and the nurse ran off and returned a few seconds later with a pair.

'They all looked at me like I was mad. I've never liked that anaesthetist. His trousers are too short. I'm always suspicious of people whose trousers are too short,' said Ruby, as Lewis poured himself a glass of wine.

'Get on with it!' said Flora, who looked as though she was about to explode. 'What happened next?'

Without a saw, Ruby improvised and, with considerable effort, used the scissors to cut through the tough cartilage that connects the ribcage to the breastplate. There was a gasp from the team as, sweating, she lifted the boy's ribcage back towards his head to expose his heart and lungs. His heart was sitting in two litres of blood. She studied the gory mess, but because his heart wasn't beating, and therefore no blood was being pumped, she couldn't see where the stab wound was. She reasoned that for him to lose so much blood so quickly it must either be in his heart or his lung. With her left hand she reached inside his chest, took hold of the root of his lungs and squeezed hard. With her other hand she took hold of his heart and squeezed. Silence. Then suddenly the boy's heart started beating.

'He's got an output,' shouted a nurse.

'Quick! Get fluids in and crossmatch blood,' shouted someone else. 'We need the cardiothoracic surgeons now!'

It was impossible for Ruby to find exactly where the stab wound was, and because she didn't know if the damaged artery or vein was in the lung or the heart, she had to keep putting pressure on both. What she did know was that if she took her hands away, he would go back into cardiac arrest. She had to stand there like that for an hour.

'I was so hungry,' said Ruby, 'that in the end I had to ask the junior doctor to get the Lion Bar out of my handbag and feed it to me. It was a little undignified, I suppose, but I think he was grateful to be of use.' It was around the time in the evening, we worked out, that Flora, Lewis, Supriya and I were drinking in the bar, wondering what had happened to Ruby.

'My phone was in my bag and I could hear I was getting text messages and phone calls. I knew they would be from you lot but, well, I had my hands full and it was rather tricky to reply without letting the boy die.' That had to be one of the best excuses for not picking up your phone I'd ever heard. Eventually the cardiothoracic surgeon arrived from the other hospital where the department was based, and the boy, with Ruby still holding his heart and lung, was rushed up to theatre.

'You literally held that boy's life in your hands,' said Flora, full of reverence.

'I thought I might still make it for drinks,' said Ruby, nonchalantly, 'but I had to go and give a statement to the police. They're treating it as attempted murder. He'd been stabbed twelve times in total – in the chest, the back and through the cheek. It's amazing he didn't die at the scene. There was a big gang of them, and just him and a female friend. Awful, isn't it?' We shook our heads silently in disgust.

'Why did they pick on him, though?' asked Flora.

'He was coming out of a gay bar,' Ruby replied.

Lewis looked at her. 'What's wrong with people?' he said quietly.

'The police told me. They cornered him and his friend, started taunting him, calling him "queer" and stuff, punched him, then knifed him. There were loads of witnesses. His friend was in A&E when I went back down and she was in absolute pieces, bawling her eyes out.'

None of us knew what to say.

'So, what happened to you tonight, then?' said Ruby, lighting a cigarette with one hand and pouring a glass of wine with the other.

Chapter 11

I knew I was shouting because the woman sitting next to me on the bus had got up and moved to another seat, and several other people were staring at me. Even the man standing opposite had removed his iPod so that he could hear what the fuss was about. 'You can't be serious?' I yelled to the person at the other end of the phone. 'Please tell me this is a joke.' I put my head into my hands.

The well-spoken man at the other end wasn't fazed. 'No, sir,' he said, clearly holding back his annoyance. 'I assure you, I'm very serious. Will you be paying by debit or credit card?'

I wasn't sure what I could say to make it clearer that I wasn't going to pay, regardless of the methods on offer.

'Well, then, you leave us no option but to call the police, sir,' he added, spitting 'sir' as though it were a new kind of insult.

Now what was I going to do? I was on my way home from work and I really didn't want to have to sort this out. It was Cassandra's fault. For one of the richest women in the world, she was bad at paying her bar bills.

In many ways she was very generous with her unparalleled wealth. Anything you asked for, she'd get it for you. She went frequently into town and spent vast amounts of money on friends and family or, indeed, on anyone she happened to meet along the way. As with so many truly wealthy people, she wasn't showy – in fact, you might have taken her for a thirty-one-year-old living in a hostel for single homeless women, receiving Disability Living Allowance. And, of course, you wouldn't be mistaken. Cassandra wasn't really a millionaire. In fact, she was deep in debt. But that didn't worry her, especially not today when it appeared she had gone into a very expensive hotel and ordered £300 worth of champagne.

The sequence of events became clear as I listened to the man at the other end of the phone. After she had finished the champagne, bought a few hotel guests some drinks and regaled them with hilarious stories of celebrities she had slept with, world leaders she had been advising and her role in the Middle East peace talks, the bill came. She had looked into her purse and, without batting an eyelid, explained that Dr Max would be paying the bill, then promptly given the telephone number for the Phoenix Project. Joy, rather baffled by what she was hearing, told the hotel manager my mobile number. I was now trying to explain to him what I should have thought was obvious: Cassandra had manic-depression and she had not been taking her medication.

Usually when people are ill, they are only too happy to receive treatment. But mania can be a strangely enjoyable experience. Cassandra was ecstatically happy, uncontrollably on top of the world. Most of us couldn't imagine the euphoria she experienced when she was ill. This was in sharp contrast to the dark depression that goes hand in hand with this illness, and which any sufferer dreads, knowing it will follow. So, of course, Cassandra resisted it when we tried to give her medication. Why would you want to swallow a tablet that would take away the best feelings you'd ever had? But the optimism that mania gives you isn't founded in reality and people get into debt. But when you're manic, you can't see that.

That was how Cassandra had become homeless. During periods of mania she would spend so outrageously that she had no money for her rent. She fell behind on her payments and eventually she was evicted onto the streets. Her landlord cleared the flat, throwing away her possessions, so when she arrived at the Phoenix Project, bedraggled and destitute, she had nothing. Haley helped her to obtain a copy of her birth certificate and apply for benefits, got her a room in a hostel and helped her to budget. Professor Pierce had put her on regular medication and visited her every week to see how she was getting on. But life in a hostel is boring when you could be a millionaire, living in the lap of luxury – even if it's only imagined. Periodically Cassandra would stop taking her medication and slip into mania.

There was something quite endearing about Cassandra, even when she was unwell. Out shopping, she would grab people and, in a conspiratorial voice, whisper, 'I'm one of the richest women in the world, you know.' Then she would press a gold bracelet or some other trinket into their hands and walk off. Underneath the delusions of grandeur she was someone who desperately wanted to be liked. How could I explain to the hotel manager that her behaviour should be seen in the context of a chronic, debilitating illness?

'Look, I cannot be held responsible for my patient's actions when I wasn't even there,' I said, getting increasingly exasperated.

'Well, I can't be held responsible for your patients if you can't keep them under control,' he replied, in a clipped tone.

'She's a person, not a rabid dog,' I snapped.

Several people looked up from their papers and glanced at me.

'Well, I'm looking at her now and that's a debatable point,' he replied.

OK, now the gloves were off. I took a deep breath. 'We can do this in one of two ways, sir,' I began, as calmly as possible. 'You can have her arrested. The police will see that she is mentally unwell and take her to hospital. That way you'll never see your money.'

By this point the other passengers on the bus were making no attempt to conceal that they were listening avidly to my conversation. The man opposite was nodding furiously in encouragement, and the woman who had moved away slunk back so that she could hear better.

The hotel manager began to protest.

'Alternatively,' I said, 'we can keep this between ourselves and not get the police involved. You can let her go and we'll find a way for Cassandra to pay what she owes you in instalments.'

'This establishment is not a charity,' began the hotel manager. 'We'll take her to court if she doesn't pay.'

I thought of the hotel residents whose lives Cassandra had briefly gatecrashed. By now they would be getting ready to go out to dinner, dripping jewels, thinking nothing of spending the GDP of a small country on food and fine wine, returning to sleep in cotton sheets spun from the hair of unicorns. Maybe I'm exaggerating, but their life was in sharp contrast to the bleak reality of Cassandra's. What she had done was wrong, but I knew that by now she would be scared and humiliated. She'd been punished enough. I'd tried reasoning with the man. Now it was time to call his bluff.

'You could take her to court,' I began lightly, 'but that would be expensive, time-consuming, and it's likely that the courts, seeing an impoverished, vulnerably housed, mentally unwell young woman, would throw the case out.' I paused for the death-blow. 'And think of the headlines: "Luxury hotel sues sick homeless woman". You'd only need a newspaper to get hold of the story, a columnist to run with it, start a campaign, and you'd have a full-blown PR disaster.'

I held my breath while I waited for his response. Silence. I could hear some muffled discussions before the manager was back. 'Of course, we always want to resolve any unfortunate incidents as amicably as possible,' he said. His tone had changed. 'May I suggest that in this particular instance the lady pays in instalments? Would you be able to oversee this?'

I relaxed. 'That sounds very reasonable,' I said and hung up. The bus passengers, still eager to know what was happening, were staring at me. On meeting my eye, they looked away and resumed what they had been doing before it had all started.

A tearful and shaking Cassandra, convinced she was about to be transported to Australia for her crimes, was duly released by the hotel's security officer, and the following day I set about trying to arrange for her to pay the bill. She came, repentant, to the Phoenix Project where Haley and I saw her. 'This is what happens when you stop taking your medication,' Haley scolded. Cassandra looked sheepish. I wrote her another prescription, which she promised to take, while Haley tried to explain that she could pay back ten pounds a week out of her benefits. Cassandra was horrified – it represented a large chunk of her weekly spending money – but realised that the time for protest was not now.

Several days later, I telephoned the hotel to arrange the repayment plan. 'Oh, no, sir. The bill has been paid,' said the receptionist. 'Another guest has settled it,' he explained.

It transpired that someone staying at the hotel had overheard the commotion. When Cassandra had left, he had taken pity on her and, in an act of remarkable generosity, had paid the bill.

I wondered what had motivated such a gesture and thought of Cassandra pressing trinkets into strangers' hands.

I telephoned Cassandra's hostel and told her the good news. She was speechless for a few moments. Then: 'I'm going to go back to the hotel and find that man and thank him.'

190

'No!' I said emphatically. 'Never, ever go back there again.'

The following day the phone rang in my office: 'Dr Pemberton, darling, there's a patient downstairs to see you,' said Joy.

'Have I got someone booked in?' I asked, puzzled: I was supposed to be going out on a visit soon.

'How should I know?' replied Joy.

'Erm, you could look in the appointments diary on your desk?' I suggested.

Joy gave a loud, exaggerated sigh. 'Well, haven't you grown up to be all demanding? Next you'll be expecting me to type your letters for you.'

'Erm, you're supposed to type my letters for me.'

'Whatever,' replied Joy. 'Do not make me click my hands in the Z formation.' She had clearly been watching too much *Jerry Springer*. 'No, darling, no one's booked in to see you,' she said, slipping out of the Bronx and back into Home Counties, 'but when you've finished you won't forget you've got to go to the ward to see Ian Hammett? Oh, and I've run out of Hobnobs, so . . .'

'No chance,' I replied, 'and, anyway, I've still got a bone to pick with you. You gave my private number to that hotel manager, didn't you? I'm going to kill you.'

'Sorry, got to dash, darling, lots of letters to type,' said Joy, laughing.

'I'll kill you,' I repeated.

'Sorry, darling, I can't hear you over the sound of my typing.' She put the phone down.

I went downstairs and there, in the waiting room, was Cassandra. 'Thank you for sorting that out,' she said, producing a package. It was a cashmere jumper.

'Oh, no!' I shouted in exasperation.

'I couldn't decide which colour to get you,' she said, 'so I got you all four.' She produced three more packages.

'Please – *please* – tell me this is a joke,' I said, and put my head into my hands.

'It's Brahms,' Ian said, staring at me intently.

I couldn't hear anything. 'What do you mean, it's Brahms?' I asked.

He stared at the floor. 'It's Brahms's fault. He stops me taking my medication,' he blurted out, as he sat, fidgeting, in his chair.

After I'd instructed Cassandra to take the cashmere jumpers back to the shop she had bought them from, then go straight home, not passing any more shops, I had come to see Ian on the ward to which he had been admitted. 'Right,' I said slowly, not sure how to respond. 'And how does he stop you taking your medication? Does he tell you not to take it?' I ventured. 'Do you hear his voice telling you what to do?'

'Of course not, he's been dead since 1897,' Ian replied. 'Anyway, he's German, and I don't speak German, so even if he did speak to me, I wouldn't understand him.'

There was a startling logic to this, which at that moment was wasted on me. I just wanted to get him to take his medication. Dr Whitfield had been trying unsuccessfully for the past two weeks and had asked me to see if I could. I'd known Ian for a while – he'd lived at the hostel, in the room next door to Talcott's, until, after six years on the housing list, he had been given a tiny studio flat. Thankfully, he didn't have a cat, because if he had and he'd wanted to swing it, he'd have encountered problems.

Shortly after he'd moved in, though, and before we could hand over his care to the local mental-health team, he'd become unwell and had had to be admitted. He was twenty-eight and had had schizophrenia since he was nineteen. Since then he had spent nearly as much time in hospital as out. He'd been on numerous medications, and countless professionals had been involved in his care. His admissions had followed a predicable course: he'd start on medication, improve, his symptoms would resolve, so that he was no longer psychotic, and he would be discharged. Within a few weeks, he'd stop taking his medication. Then it was just a countdown until he was readmitted to hospital. Typically he became paranoid. He heard voices constantly when he was unwell, and believed that the television was sending him messages and interfering with his thoughts. 'Keep taking the medication and you won't need to come into hospital,' I said, trying to convince him.

'I know, Doctor,' he said, looking up at me after several minutes of staring at the floor.

Over the months I had been doing this job, I had come to understand that things were rarely black and white. On the streets, among those at the hinterland of society and the extremes of human experience, the complex, multiple shades of grey are shown in their full splendour. It might be comforting to think that for every problem there is an answer, for every ailment a cure. But sometimes the cure can cause as many problems as the ailment. In reality, a careful balancing act is required. Sometimes there is no simple answer, no magic bullet.

It transpired that it was indeed Brahms that was stopping Ian taking his medication. Or, rather, it was his love of Brahms, and indeed Elgar. Ian played the cello. His brother was a music teacher and his sister a professional musician. Reading through his notes, it was clear that, from an early age, Ian had shown a stunning gift for music. But just after he had begun his degree he was hit by the first symptoms of his illness. He didn't complete it, although he had never stopped playing the cello. Until now. No medication is without potential side effects and, tragically for Ian, the anti-psychotic medication that treated the symptoms of his schizophrenia gave him an adverse effect called akathisia. This is a type of the 'extra-pyramidal side effect' that Flora had inadvertently encountered, but of a very severe nature. Put simply, it's restlessness, and in Ian it manifested itself as a constant, crippling inability to keep his legs still.

When he played his cello, he lost himself in his own world and forgot his illness. It gave him a connection with the rest of his family who had to contend with the extremes of his illness and couldn't recognise the chaotic, dishevelled man he became at times. It gave him purpose and meaning in his life. He had failed to hold on to any other personal possessions, but he had always kept his cello with him and now I understood why, but because of the medication, he couldn't play it. That, he explained, was why he never took his medication after he was discharged from hospital.

194

While Cassandra stopped taking hers because she enjoyed her illness, he stopped because he hated the cost of being well. I wondered why he'd never told anyone this before.

'Because doctors wouldn't understand. They just want to treat me with tablets, but I always figured I'd rather be ill and able to play the cello than well and without my music,' he said slowly. Without the medication he couldn't function properly, but if he took it he lost the one thing he loved. It was an impossible situation. I knew, and so did he, that he needed to take his medication. But I also grasped that it meant making an unbearable sacrifice. 'I know you're right, Doctor,' he said eventually.

Success. But as I signed the prescription and prepared to tell Dr Whitfield the good news, all I could think was that I was depriving him of his *raison d'être*. It was a painfully hollow victory.

'I'll take it this time. It's pointless trying to resist,' Ian said.

This should have been music to my ears, but it wasn't.

Tentatively I put my foot on the first stair.

'You'll be careful, Doctor, won't you?' came a voice from the sitting room.

I placed the other foot carefully on the next. The floorboard creaked and I froze. I waited a few moments and gingerly went up a few more, hardly daring to breathe.

After I'd left Ian, Kevin had phoned as I was walking back to the office. He had a request. Surprisingly, it didn't involve Joy and a packet of Hobnobs. It was unusual because it involved seeing a patient in a house. A real, proper, four-walls-and-a-roof house. This was quite exciting: I was used to seeing patients under park benches (that's the patients, not me), in alleys or stations. The nearest I ever got to a house was a hostel, which just wasn't the same.

I wondered, as I walked to the address where I would meet Kevin, if they'd offer me tea in a proper china cup with a saucer instead of the polystyrene ones I was now so accustomed to.

I reached the landing and took a moment to plan my next move. I looked behind me and saw a photograph framed on the wall. It was of a family sitting on a beach: pebbles, grey skies and drizzle. Ah, the great British holiday, I thought. They were eating ice cream and laughing. I recognised the adults sitting at either side of their two children as the parents who, at that moment, were downstairs with Kevin. There was a boy of perhaps twelve in the picture, with a towel wrapped round him. That must be Tom. I stared at his face and wondered when it had begun to go wrong. Probably a few years after that photograph was taken.

I heard a noise from the bedroom across the landing and made my way over to it. The door was ajar. I peered inside and was hit by the rank smell of urine and faeces. It was unbearably hot and stuffy. 'Hello, Tom. Are you in here?' I asked softly, into the darkness.

I heard a rustle. Slowly, as my eyes became used to the dark, I realised that the patterns on the wall were smeared excrement. The carpet was peppered with cigarette burns, and shredded newspaper.

196

I could just make out someone crouching by the bed. 'Hello. I'm a doctor. Your parents are very worried about you so they asked me to come and talk to you,' I said. Nothing. Then a sudden scream, and something hurtled out of the darkness and smashed against the wall behind me. I left hurriedly and closed the door as something else smashed. There was thumping, more screaming, a loud crash, then silence again.

I went downstairs and back to his parents, who were sitting on the sofa.

'Any luck?' Kevin asked.

'No,' I replied. 'He's not going to talk to me. We're going to have to section him and get the police to bring him into hospital.'

Tom's mother began to cry while his father comforted her. 'It's for the best,' he said, in a low, hoarse whisper.

A slow and insidious trajectory had resulted in Tom's condition. His parents weren't sure when it had started, but they agreed that, soon after he had taken his GCSEs, things had begun to change. When his father had caught him smoking cannabis in his room, Tom had threatened to move out.

I wrote down everything they told me, but it was a story I'd heard so many times.

He had started using skunk, a stronger form of cannabis, and things had really gone downhill. Tom rarely came out of his room. He became volatile and aggressive. His mother heard him talking to himself and crying late at night. In desperation they called the GP, but then Tom vanished. Paranoid that his family were poisoning him, he ended up on the streets. His parents searched for him day and night. His sister printed posters and stuck them up everywhere she could think of.

They didn't know it, but Kevin had already found Tom, wandering around the station. He had arranged for Tom to go into emergency hostel accommodation for a few nights while a proper assessment could be arranged with Professor Pierce. Before that could happen, Tom had gone missing again. He wouldn't agree to come into hospital – which, clearly, he desperately needed – but he evaded any attempt to section him and bring him in against his will. Whenever Kevin tracked him down, Tom would move on.

Eventually he went home briefly, and his parents found Kevin's contact details in his coat pocket. His father had telephoned Kevin directly and, rather than the formal route of a GP referring Tom to the local community mental-health team, Kevin felt it was best for all concerned if he and I went out straight away.

The wards are littered with similar examples of lives wrecked, sometimes for a short time, sometimes permanently. Since training in medicine I have seen dozens of people who have become psychotic after using cannabis, and the number has increased as the stronger forms, such as skunk, have become more widely available. The libertarian in me thinks that people should be free to make choices about what they do to themselves, which includes using cannabis. Then I remember people like Tom, who aren't making informed decisions about the risks because few ever witness the true horrors of what skunk can do, the way it can fracture someone's mind, strip them of a future, and devastate a family. The lives it ruins aren't on display for everyone to see. They're locked away in psychiatric hospitals, or shut away in homes while parents wring their hands and doctors wonder when it all went wrong.

That evening, I arrived home tired and in need of a drink. Ruby had beaten me to it and cracked open a bottle. 'Look! I thought of you immediately,' she exclaimed, before I'd even sat down. She was waving a newspaper in my face.

I read the headline: 'Sexually Transmitted Diseases On The Increase'. 'Why did you think of me? What do you know that I don't?' I asked.

'Not that. *That,*' she said, pointing to an article about the trial of a man with schizophrenia who had escaped from a secure psychiatric unit and murdered someone. She poured herself more wine and took a drag on her cigarette. 'I don't know how you do that job. Doesn't that sort of news story scare you?' She exhaled a thin plume of smoke. 'There's no way you'd get me doing it. Give me a road-traffic accident over a psychotic person any day.'

Ruby was practical. She liked getting her hands dirty, people coming to her *in extremis* so that she could put them right. She didn't care about the gore, the blood and guts: she liked the immediacy of working in trauma surgery. She wanted clear, defined outcomes from her job: they were bleeding and now they were not; they had a fractured leg, and now they could walk again. There was none of this in my job. The end points were nebulous and blurred. There was no dramatic resolution to intervention, no guaranteed cure.

This still bothered me, although I had begun to enjoy the gradual building of a relationship with a patient, trying to understand someone in their entirety, hearing their story. Flora had decided she didn't like sick people. That was unfortunate as it's an occupational hazard for a doctor to meet them. But she had found possibly the only branch of medicine in which the patients are not necessarily sick: obstetrics. She had to do gynaecology as well, but the depressing aspects of this were offset by the excitement of delivering babies. In this field, tragedies were infrequent enough to mean that she wasn't emotionally drained when they happened and, for the most part, she loved being there to make each woman's experience of giving birth as pleasant as possible. After only a week in the job she had returned home with two goals: first, to become an obstetrician and, second, never to have children. 'It's like a car crash down there once it's all over,' she had said, swallowing hard. 'It's a miracle but, God, it's a painful, messy one.' Flora was on-call tonight, no doubt making coochie-coo noises to newborn babies on the maternity wards as we spoke and nibbling rusks surreptitiously in the laundry cupboard between Caesarean sections.

'Doesn't it ever scare you, working with the sorts of people you do?' asked Ruby, as she started on another glass of wine. It was Friday night and she was going for it.

I thought about this. I have a low threshold for being scared. Never mind hiding behind the sofa throughout an episode of *Doctor Who*, I've been known to reach for a cushion during *Murder, She Wrote*. You'd imagine, therefore, given the bad press that those with mental illness attract, that I'd be a jabbering bag of nerves working with them day in, day out. Clearly, I was going to get murdered and they'd eat my liver with a glass of Chianti. But, of course, that wasn't the case. None of the patients wore Hannibal Lecter masks and I had yet to bump into Jodie Foster. Rather than fear, my prevailing feeling was of sadness at how mental illness could destroy lives. When I was out with friends, they stared, wide-eyed, when I told them about my patients at the Phoenix Project. 'Isn't it scary with all those nutters?' they'd ask. No, was the simple answer. It was many things – such as frustrating and sad – but not scary. I thought of Ian and the slow, insidious way in which his life had been dismantled by his mental illness. Even when someone was acutely unwell, like Tom, they were far more scared of you than you were of them.

But the image of axe-wielding maniacs is pervasive in our society, and cases reported in the media of people with schizophrenia murdering others do nothing to dispel this. Such stories are always tricky. Of course they're news and therefore it's understandable they're reported. But they help to fan the flames of fear in the general public that mentally ill people, especially schizophrenics, are dangerous. It's easy to forget that what makes such stories newsworthy is the very fact that the incidents are so rare. In fact, people with schizophrenia do pose a significant danger – to themselves: one in ten commits suicide. The isolation they experience as a result of the stigma of mental illness is thought to be one of the main contributing factors. Put like this, we, the general public, pose a far greater risk to schizophrenics than they do to us. I thought of Ian, Barry and Mr Allsop. Their lives had been irreparably altered by their illness. They evoked in me many feelings, but fear was not one of them.

The risk of being killed by someone with mental illness is about the same as that of being struck by lightning. Far more people are killed as a result of domestic violence, yet we don't all get jittery when someone gets married. And although drunk people don't provoke the same level of fear in the public that schizophrenics do, it's much safer to live next to an asylum than to a pub: intoxication is implicated in far more homicides than mental illness. Think about that next time you sit down with a nice glass of Chianti.

Chapter 12

'We're all going to die,' Bruce screamed, as he rocked back and forth.

Joy slapped the back of his head. 'Shut up, man, you're driving me mad.'

'I'm thirsty,' said Tammy, for the hundredth time.

'I need the toilet,' added Rachel.

This, I concluded, was hell. As a social experiment it was interesting: take a random assortment of people, including a doctor, two nurses, two receptionists and two drug addicts, lock them into a room with no windows for several hours and see what happens.

'Look,' I said, increasingly exasperated, 'the police will be outside by now and this will be over soon. Now, please, everyone, just stay calm.' I looked pointedly at Bruce.

'This is like one of those zombie movies where everyone's trapped and they have to eat each other because they're starving and then they become no better than the zombies outside,' said Bruce, hysterically.

I looked at Joy, who kindly obliged and slapped him again. There was a time and a place for concerns regarding bullying in the workplace, and trapped in a room on a Friday afternoon while an acutely psychotic woman was on the rampage in the corridor outside was neither the time nor the place for them.

I consulted my watch. We'd only been in there for forty minutes and already people were getting cabin fever.

'Let's play I Spy,' said Amy.

No one responded to this suggestion but she continued undeterred.

'I spy with my little eye something beginning with . . .' she paused '. . . M.'

'Murderers?' suggested Bruce, staring at us. 'All of us, potential murderers. It's in situations like this where society breaks down and we revert to our animalistic urges.'

'No,' said Amy, 'and, anyway, technically that should be PM, for potential murderers.'

'Is it Marmite?' suggested Rachel. 'I really fancy some Marmite. Or Maltesers.'

'Mmm, yeah, Maltesers,' interrupted Tony, who had been dozing on a chair. 'Has anyone got any?'

'No,' snapped Amy. There was little in the room, actually, except a few chairs and tables.

'I'm thirsty,' repeated Tammy. I began to wonder if Bruce was being so alarmist after all: I could happily have throttled her if she'd said that just once more.

There was silence for a few moments. 'Marmoset,' said Tony.

'What?' said Amy. 'Why the hell would there be a marmoset in the room?'

'Oh,' said Tony, 'does it have to be in the room?'

I sighed. 'We give up,' I announced.

'Magazine,' she said, pointing to a leaflet on herpes that was lying on one of the tables.

'That's not a magazine,' I protested. 'It's a pamphlet.'

'OK,' Amy said. 'I spy with my little eye something beginning with P.' She sat back in her chair.

I wasn't being paid enough for this, I decided.

The day had started unremarkably. I was actually supposed to be working at the Phoenix Project that afternoon. I had sat on Joy's desk while she filed her nails and regaled me with stories of her latest run-in with her local council. She was always having run-ins with the council – or with people behind the counter at the post office, or her MP. In fact, with just about anyone in authority who crossed her path. Writing letters of complaint was her hobby, and she took pride in the large volume of correspondence she had generated over the years. It was a shame she didn't take such an interest in the letters I gave her to type, especially as it was her job to take an interest in them. Her complaints were never financially driven: she didn't look for compensation. She aimed for deference. She liked nothing better than returning to a shop where she had complained to the manager and watching everyone scuttle round her as though she were royalty. The binmen, she told me with pride, now bowed when she walked past. I wondered if they weren't doing this with a hint of irony, but she seemed to think they wouldn't dare. 'I'll write to the waste-disposal manager, though, just in case,' she said, with a frown.

Aside from writing letters, the other thing that took up Joy's time was eating. Before she would consider typing for someone in the office they had to supply her with a packet of biscuits, and if it involved an Excel spreadsheet, they'd better be chocolate-covered. I had asked Joy to do some photocopying, which she enjoyed because she had to leave the office and use the machine in the drug-dependency unit next door. The photocopier at the Phoenix Project had been broken since I had begun work there. I suspected that the only reason it remained unfixed was to give Joy an excuse to go out. Unlike most of her administration duties, photocopying was the only one that didn't necessitate extensive pleading with her. Of course, it did take her half the day. No one was quite sure why, but once when I was in McDonald's, waiting for a patient, I saw someone who looked suspiciously like Joy duck behind a chair and make a run for the exit before I could say hello.

Joy had to do some photocopying and I had to sign some prescriptions, so we went to the drug-dependency unit together. I followed Joy into the downstairs office to check my post and almost immediately heard shouting coming from the corridor where the interview rooms were. A few patients were sitting in the waiting room, unconcerned. I turned to Amy, who was at the reception desk. 'Who's shouting?' I asked. 'Is everything OK, do you think?'

Amy nodded. 'Yeah, don't worry. It's just Georgia. She came in for her prescription but was really weird so Tony took her in there to see what was up.'

'Shouldn't we check he's OK?' I wondered.

'Oh, you know her, she's going through one of her funny spells. She's been using crack again – it always sends her a bit loopy.' Bruce was milling about, clearly miffed that Joy was using *his* photocopier.

Suddenly we heard a loud crash. It had come from the interview rooms. Within seconds Amy was on her feet and rushing through the waiting room to be met by Tony, who was racing towards her. 'She's smashing the place up! She's like a bull in a china shop!' he yelled, hurtling into the office. 'Except she was smashing furniture, not china, because we don't have any china in there for health and safety reasons – and also there's just no need . . .' he twittered, trying to catch his breath.

It was then that our attention turned to the patients, who were still sitting, somewhat bemused, in the waiting room. 'We need to evacuate the building. It's not safe with her like that,' said Amy. Usually Sister Stein would take control of a situation like this, but she was on leave. Amy sounded the alarm, which was linked to the local police station, and we went into the waiting room. 'We're evacuating the building,' she explained, as calmly as she could. But before anyone could move, Georgia lumbered into the waiting room. I admit that this time I was a little scared. She was a formidable size and was carrying a chair. Several patients got up and left. Rachel, now eight months pregnant, stayed in her seat. We edged towards the exit, while Georgia swung the chair. She smashed it against the wall and it fell to pieces. At this point Tammy emerged from the lavatory. Momentarily Georgia was distracted and Amy took the opportunity to grab Rachel and usher her towards the office where the others were huddled. Tammy, blissfully unaware of what was happening, strolled past Georgia, glancing at the broken chair.

The next thing that happened shaped the following two hours. Georgia charged towards us, waving a piece of chair. We scattered and Georgia went into the lobby, positioning herself between us and the front door. Tony edged forward and shut the door into the waiting room, thus separating us off from Georgia.

Everyone breathed a sigh of relief.

Georgia started banging on the window pane with the broken chair. 'It's OK,' said Bruce, who until this point had remained very calm. 'It's toughened glass. She'll never break it.'

There was a horrendous crash. Georgia had smashed her way through the glass.

Pandemonium broke out. In our panic, we ran past the fire escape towards the interview rooms, hotly pursued by Georgia.

That was how we had found ourselves trapped in a windowless room at the back of the clinic going stir-crazy. 'It's the only room down here with a lock on the door,' said Amy, sulking when we realised there was no way out. 'I thought it would be safe in here.'

'You could have led us out of the fire escape in the waiting room,' said Bruce, irritably. 'I think I'm getting one of my migraines.'

'Well, you didn't have to follow me. You could have taken charge, couldn't you?' retorted Amy.

'OK, everyone keep calm. Amy pressed the alarm so the police will be here soon,' I said.

Joy had her mobile with her and was already talking to them. Suddenly everyone shrieked. Georgia was peering through the little window in the door. She began hitting it with the broken chair.

'It's OK—' began Bruce.

'Let me guess, it's toughened glass?' interrupted Joy. 'Oh, now I feel much better, because the last time you said that everything turned out so well, didn't it?'

'I'm thirsty,' said Tammy, for the first time.

Forty minutes later, we had established that the police were considering this a hostage situation. The problem was, Georgia couldn't be negotiated with. She had a developed drug-induced psychosis, which was why she had gone on the rampage. Like all psychoses, this manifested itself as a loss of contact with reality, associated hallucinations, abnormal beliefs, paranoia and disorganised thoughts. It had been brought on in Georgia by crack. It is well known among the patients that one of crack's side effects is paranoia. A number of times I had sat with patients who had just smoked it and watched their eyes dart furtively about the room as though they were being watched. Users often report hearing voices. Usually at this stage they stop taking it for a few days and the symptoms dissipate. But not Georgia. She would continue to use it even when it was clearly sending her insane. She had been admitted to hospital several times with drug-induced psychosis, sometimes requiring sedation. Over a few days and with medication, she would get better and be discharged. But this time she had become convinced that the drug-dependency unit was a government organisation that had samples of her tissue, which they were using to clone people. When Tony had tried to reason with her and suggested she might need to go back into hospital, she became convinced that he was part of the conspiracy and had been trying to poison her with the methadone.

It was when Tony was explaining this to us all that I discovered I had lice. It's never a welcome diagnosis, not least when you're stuck in a room full of people with no way out. I had been scratching the back of my neck while Tony elaborated on exactly how he had escaped from Georgia when I felt a sharp pain. When I looked at my hand, there was a speck of blood on my finger. I felt along my hairline and found something odd stuck at the base of a hair. I tugged at it until it came away. I brought my hand down and there, in front of me, was a little creature. It was a while before I realised it was a louse and unlikely to be alone. I was immediately itchy everywhere. I spent the next minute scratching frantically all over my body, and the more I scratched, the more I became convinced I could feel them crawling over me. 'I think I've got lice,' I whispered to Amy.

'Ooh, what have you been up to, you naughty boy?' She raised an eyebrow.

'Not that sort. Body lice. I must have caught them off one of my patients.'

She was scratching too now. 'We've got stuff in the clinic room for it. You can take some if we ever get out of here alive.'

'Don't worry,' I said, putting a hand on her knee. 'The police will get her out any minute.'

'Do you mind taking your hand off my leg?' she said, and shivered.

I resumed scratching.

There was more crashing from outside. Rachel and

Tammy clung to each other. Joy sat filing her nails, apparently unperturbed.

'Don't do that,' said Tony, pointing to Joy's nail file. 'We might be able to use it to escape.'

'Do you actually work here or are you one of the patients on drugs?' asked Joy, in her usual acerbic tone. 'It's an emery board, for God's sake, not a pickaxe. What do you think this is? Colditz?'

'I need the toilet,' said Rachel, who was sitting behind me. 'The baby's pressing on me bladder.' She shifted uncomfortably in her chair.

Any mention of her baby made me wince. Sister Stein had recently attended a meeting with Social Services and it seemed increasingly likely that the baby would be taken away from Rachel and placed with a foster-family.

'When's it due?' asked Tammy.

'A month today,' replied Rachel.

'I bet you're excited. Babies are so adorable, aren't they?' said Tammy.

'Yeah, I'm so looking forward to seeing his little face.'

I sank lower in my chair, convinced she was doing this deliberately to torture me.

'I got a new buggy last weekend – it's wicked, you should see it,' she continued.

'They're pricy, ain't they? How'd you afford a new one?' asked Tammy, innocently.

Rachel giggled. 'I got my ways,' she said.

I wondered what they were.

She had always been reticent about discussing how she funded her drug addiction. I had been rather surprised to learn when I first started work there that most of the patients were on benefits: I understood that if the state didn't give them money they would find enough for drugs in one way or another but it seemed rather strange that my taxes were used to fund an illegal activity.

'You're not turning Tory on me, are you?' Ruby had asked, when I'd discussed it with her.

'It's not that. It just seems, well, not right somehow. I mean, we see so many people who really need help from the state because of illness and disease through no fault of their own.'

'You can't go down that route,' said Ruby. 'Otherwise we wouldn't treat smokers and drinkers.' She had offered me a cigarette to illustrate her point. 'Where do you draw the line? What about people who injure themselves doing sport? Isn't it their fault they got hurt? Maybe we should only treat people who sit at home and are totally risk averse.'

I knew what she was saying, but it still didn't seem right. 'I don't know what the solution is,' I said.

'They employ you to get them off drugs and into jobs. You're the solution,' Ruby said, with a smile.

But many of my patients spent vast sums of money on their addiction and had to steal despite the benefits. Not all of them were like Fergal and Anthony, with their moral code of conduct.

I continued to eavesdrop on Rachel and Tammy's conversation. I sat daily with people who not only used drugs but stole, burgled and mugged people in order to do so. I tried not to think about this because being judgemental was counterproductive, but it was a sore point for me at that time, not only because of my near-death experience and Barry's injuries, which were still healing, but because my grandparents had been burgled only the weekend before. At the same time, Rachel was buying her new buggy using money she had undoubtedly got through unpleasant means. OK, so my grandparents lived miles away and it wasn't their money she was spending, but that was hardly the point.

I'd been out for a drink with Flora when my mum phoned. 'Something awful's happened,' she said.

'Don't tell me the dog's been sick on your laptop again. I keep telling you not to leave it on the floor,' I replied, rolling my eyes.

Flora had laughed.

'No, that's not it, although she has thrown up on it again. Your gran's been burgled. She's quite upset. I'm going over tomorrow but it would be nice if you'd give them a call.' She paused, and I guessed what was coming next. 'I know you're busy but . . .'

It was a trick of my mum's not to complete a sentence when she wanted me to do something: she made me guess what she was going to say so that it sounded as though it was my idea. I fell for it every time. 'Would I go over and help?' I suggested.

'Oh, what a lovely idea. You are a good boy.'

I put the phone down and finished my drink, then went to the station. By the time I got there it was late. My grandmother opened the door. She'd obviously been crying. I hugged her and followed her into the lounge. The place had been ransacked: broken glass on the floor, drawers opened, their contents spilled everywhere. She'd been told not to touch anything until the police arrived, but that had been hours ago so she had decided to clear up. 'They never catch them anyway, do they?' she said, with a shrug.

'You've got to write down everything you notice missing,' I said, although of course she had already started doing this – 'The country didn't win a war by being shoddy at administration,' she was wont to remark . . . usually when I complained about not having done my self-assessment tax return.

They had taken all the usual things: the TV, the DVD player, some cash from a pot on the mantelpiece, a camera, my grandmother's mobile phone ('Why have a mobile phone and leave it at home?' I wanted to ask, but thought better of it). They'd taken her engagement ring, which had belonged to my great-grandmother, some jewellery that my grandfather had bought her over the years, a pair of pearl earrings that her sister had given her before she died, and so on. She'd had little of worth, but what she'd had, they had taken. 'They're just objects, I suppose,' said Gran, stoically. Clearly they had been after things they could convert quickly into cash as they'd left behind a valuable clock and an antique side table that had been in the family for generations. 'It's just not nice to think that someone else has been in your house, touching things.' They'd smashed the window to get in and the dog, who was practically blind and deaf, and as good a guard dog as a wet flannel, had walked on the shards of glass, cut his paws and bled all over the house.

'Oh, they've taken that graduation photo of yours,' said Gran, as we tidied up. 'I expect they were after the frame.'

My grandfather was upstairs.

'I'll carry on here. You go up and see him,' said Gran. Upstairs, there was a similarly chaotic scene in the bedroom. My grandfather was sitting on the bed, looking at a photo of himself and Gran. Every time I saw them they seemed frailer, and he had a large dressing on his forehead where a benign skin growth had been removed that day at the hospital. His hands shook as he held out the photo. 'Look what I've found,' he said. 'It was on the floor, just there. I haven't looked at it for years.'

They had been in their twenties. He was wearing shorts and I smiled at his knobbly knees. He had an arm round my gran. 'I was about your age when it was taken,' he said.

There was a brief silence and then he raged, 'How dare they? Who do they think they are, coming in here and taking our stuff?' He coughed.

'It's all right, Granddad, we'll straighten everything out,' I said, attempting to pacify him.

'It's not all right. Little sods – after money for drugs, no doubt.'

I suspected he was right. They would probably only get a few hundred pounds for the stuff they had taken and no professional burglar would have bothered with such small pickings. But what they had taken was priceless to my grandparents and I was furious to think of their belongings being flogged off dirt cheap by some crack-head so they could get their next fix. My grandparents weren't rich. They had worked hard all their lives, saved up for the things they wanted, never hurt anyone.

Eventually the police arrived, but there was little they could do now. They sat down with my grandparents for a bit and took details, then went on their way.

I stayed the night and, in the morning, resumed the clear-up until my mum and sister arrived to take over. On the train home I thought about my patients and wondered which ones were funding their habits in the same way. That was the thing about illegal drugs: they affected everyone. The lives of the patients I saw spread out like tentacles and touched everyone in different ways. We constantly paid the price for other people's addiction, either directly by being mugged or having our property stolen, or indirectly through banks or shops that passed on to us the cost of fraud and theft. But maybe troubled individuals are the product of a troubled society. All the time I came up against such questions to which there were no ready answers.

I gradually became aware that Rachel and Tammy were whispering and strained to hear what they were saying. 'Two brown and one white,' said Tammy.

'Sure,' replied Rachel. 'I'll drop them round later.'

Suddenly I was filled with rage: not only had Rachel been using drugs throughout her pregnancy but she was supplying Tammy with them. She was making her money from dealing. Her own child would be born an addict, and she was stopping Tammy getting clean. I thought back to when I'd first met Tammy and the high hopes I'd had for her to be the one I saved. Now, in the very place where people were supposed to be getting better, Rachel was selling drugs under my nose. There was nothing I could say or do, but in a moment of spite I was pleased that Rachel's baby would be taken away. She didn't deserve happiness.

I took a deep breath. If Tammy hadn't got the drugs from Rachel she'd have found another dealer. I was angry with Rachel, but maybe that was a reflection of how angry she was with herself. Deep down, no one wanted her life, least of all Rachel. No drug addict wanted the life they'd created for themselves. I'd learnt that much.

The situation came to an abrupt and unexpected end. 'Right,' said Joy. 'It's five o'clock.' She stood up. 'Well, come on, then, I'm getting my hair done tonight and I can't be late.' Then, to our horror and amazement, she went over to the door and opened it.

'No!' screamed Amy.

Joy didn't look back.

'"Cowards die many times before their deaths: the valiant never taste of death but once",' shouted Bruce, now back to his usual self as he jumped to his feet. '*Julius Caesar*, Act Two, scene two,' he called back to us, as he made a dash for the door.

We got up and hurried to peer out and watch what happened. I was just in time to see Joy, in one smooth, perfectly co-ordinated move, grapple Georgia to the floor at the end of the corridor and sit on her. Georgia was so stunned that she simply lay there, blinking. Bruce edged past them and, within a few seconds, the police were there. 'Well, don't just stand around. I've got better things to do than act as a human paperweight,' Joy said to one of the officers. They moved forward and restrained Georgia.

'Why didn't you do that to start with?' asked Amy.

Joy shrugged. 'I'd have had to go back to the office,' she said. Then she yelped. 'Oh, my God.' Her face twisted.

'What? What is it?' Amy went to her.

'I've broken a bloody nail,' she said, holding her finger aloft.

I bet she writes a complaint letter about it, I thought.

Everyone left the clinic but I had something on my mind. Or, rather, on my person. A lot of things, I imagined. I went to the clinic room, found the anti-louse lotion and dashed off to the lavatory to douse myself in it. It smelt revolting, but I didn't care. 'Die! Die!' I said, as I rubbed it all over me.

'You won't believe what's happened to me today,' I said, as I walked in through the front door. I was met by silence. 'Hello? Anyone home?' I called. I heard a noise in the kitchen and went in to find Ruby sitting in the dark on her own. 'What are you doing in here with the light off?' I said, turning it on. Ruby's head was in her hands, but then she looked up. Her eyes were puffy, her face red and wet. 'What's wrong?' I asked, horrified. 'What's happened?'

I had obviously caught her off guard because she tried quickly to compose herself. 'I thought you were getting the train to your gran's this evening to see how she was,' she said, as she wiped her face.

'Yeah, but I got a bit delayed at work so I'll go in the morning. But what's happened?'

Ruby sighed. 'It's nothing. It's just me being stupid.' She lit a cigarette and inhaled deeply.

'Where's Flora?' I asked.

'She's on-call. I didn't think you'd be back tonight so I was just sitting here having a think.'

'You should have called me if you were upset. Now, tell me what's happened,' I said, sitting down.

218

'I just . . .' began Ruby, and hesitated. 'I just sometimes think maybe we shouldn't interfere.'

'Look, if this is about Flora's budgie escaping out of that window, nobody blames you. That was ages ago anyway. She's forgotten about it now and I'm sure he's made a lovely home in some park somewhere.' I wasn't at all sure of this and suspected that he had met his maker in the shape of next door's cat.

Ruby shook her head. 'Of course I don't mean that.' She shifted in her seat. 'Sometimes I think maybe we do more harm than good – as doctors, I mean. That we meddle in things and set off a whole chain of events that are out of our control.' She lifted the cigarette towards her mouth but left it resting on her lip, suspended, as she thought. 'I went to see that boy – you know, Joel, the one who got stabbed.'

The story of how she had saved the boy's life by cutting through his breastplate had spread and she was now a minor celebrity in doctors' circles. She was nearly up there with Dr Hilary Jones.

'I knew I shouldn't have gone. I knew it would be a mistake. The whole point about trauma surgery is you stabilise the patient, save their life and don't look back.'

'What happened? Wasn't he pleased to see you?' I asked.

'He's paralysed. He can't even use a wheelchair. He can't feed himself, he can't do anything. He's like a vegetable, except it's worse than that because he knows what's happening.'

'Why? You saved him; I thought he was OK?' I asked slowly.

219

'He hasn't left intensive care yet. He's had meningitis. The knife they stabbed him with was dirty.' She gave a brief, hollow laugh. 'I suppose you don't think about sterilising the knife before you stab someone.' She took a drag on her cigarette. 'One of the stab wounds went into his spinal cord and the infection travelled up to his brain.' It had left him brain damaged and paralysed.

For a few moments I didn't reply. Ruby was usually so strong and self-assured, and had counselled me many times about patients who had needed my help, and now I wanted to say the right thing. 'It's not your fault, Rubes. You saved his life. You weren't to know what would happen. You're blaming yourself for something that was totally out of your control. You couldn't have just left him there to die.'

'Yeah, but look what I've condemned him to now. What kind of life have I saved for him? I should have just let him go, not been so determined.' She looked at me. 'You do these things, you bring people back from the brink of death, but I wonder if it's always in the patient's best interests. We don't think about that in an emergency. There's no nice little sit-down chat with the family and cups of tea like on TV. There's no medical ethicist on hand and group discussion, like at medical school. It happens so fast and you just act. You make a split-second judgement – is it worth saving this person? – and he has to deal with the consequences for the rest of his life.' She got up, filled the kettle and plugged it in.

'He's only twenty-two, Max. He'll have decades living like that. You know what it's like. He'll keep getting pneumonia and they'll pump him full of antibiotics, he'll be in and out of hospital, round-the-clock carers, no dignity, no independence. And if I hadn't been walking past when they wheeled him in he'd have died in A&E and it would all be over.' The kettle had boiled and she got two mugs from the cupboard. 'It just seems so pointless somehow. You think you're doing good, yet it turns out the opposite.' She finished making the tea and walked over to the table.

'Ruby,' I said, 'you did your best and you weren't to know. The people who are responsible for how things have turned out are the people who stabbed him. Not you. It's their fault. Blame them.'

She put the tea on the table. 'I don't really want tea,' she said eventually. 'Do you fancy going for a drink?'

'Yeah, come on,' I said, and stood up.

We left the flat and walked along the road. I put my arm round her.

'How was your day at work?' she asked after a while, looking at me and smiling. 'And what's that awful smell?'

'Well . . .'

A few seconds later she pushed my arm away and began to scratch.

Chapter 13

'You've got to prepare yourself for the worst,' said Lynne. 'If he was out for the past few nights, he probably . . .' Her voice trailed off.

Professor Pierce said, 'I think what Lynne is trying to say is that it's possible he's died.'

There was an awkward silence, which was broken by Joy opening a packet of biscuits. Professor Pierce looked at her and shook his head. 'Sorry,' she murmured, and pulled a face when he'd turned away. She leant forward. 'They're luxury, darling,' she said with a nod, as she offered me the packet, having taken one for herself, of course. 'Look, they've got chunks of real Belgian chocolate in them.'

'I'm OK, thanks all the same,' I said.

Kevin leant forward to try and help himself but Joy snatched them away. She took another and pushed the whole thing pointedly into her mouth. She narrowed her eyes and did a Cheshire-cat grin, rubbing her stomach.

Kevin began to protest and Joy gave in. 'There you go, darling,' she said, handing him one. 'Now you owe me.'

Kevin looked slightly perturbed, as well he might: Joy kept close tabs on those who owed her favours. One biscuit roughly translated into a back massage or unlimited requests for cups of coffee. With interest rates like that, Joy was more the office loan-shark than the secretary.

As diverting as Joy's antics could be, none of this was making me feel any better. Rarely had a patient consumed my thoughts in the way that Patrick had lately. He had turned up at the Phoenix Project three days ago. That morning Joy had arrived, muffin in hand, to open the office and found him squatting by the front door, shivering. She had let him in, sat him down in one of the interview rooms and even made him a cup of tea. He had been wandering around all night looking for somewhere to stay and had heard from people at the station that we might be able to help. 'Poor little thing. He'll catch his death out there. He looks so innocent, like an angel,' she said.

I didn't believe in angels, especially in this line of work. I went down to see him.

Patrick was twenty-two, quiet and reserved, with striking features and wispy, blond hair. He made only fleeting eye-contact and rocked on his chair when he spoke to me. I suspected he had mild learning difficulties and certainly wouldn't survive on the streets for long. He didn't have any family: he had watched his dad kill his mum when he was eight, and since then had spent most of his life in institutions. When he was sixteen he was sent to a young-offenders unit after he had been involved in a robbery during which someone had been shot. He had only recently been released. He had been sleeping outside for the past month but now it was too cold for him. The previous night he hadn't slept at all. He had a chest infection and his whole body shook when he coughed. It would take weeks to get him into a hostel but he was so totally alone, so desperate and lost that I couldn't bear to turn him away.

'Wait here,' I said, and went back upstairs to find a list of shelters where he could go that night.

'We'll have to find him a place in a hostel,' said Haley, who had just arrived.

'I know, but that'll take too long. He needs somewhere tonight,' I said, and went back downstairs.

In the interview room, Patrick took the piece of paper. 'Try this shelter,' I said, circling the first one. 'Our address and phone number are at the top if there are any problems.'

He stared at it. 'Which way do I go?' he asked. 'I don't really know the city.'

'The directions are written on there,' I said, pointing and reading them aloud to him. 'Come back tomorrow and we'll try to find something more permanent for you,' I said, as I showed him out. That was the last time I had seen him. The following day Patrick didn't come back.

When I was young I used to peer out of the window on winter mornings, my nose pressed to the pane, and pray for snow. Snow is great – but only when it's combined with roaring fires, black-and-white films on TV and buttered toast, all of which are in short supply when you're homeless. The day after I'd seen Patrick there had been reports of plummeting temperatures, and severe weather warnings were broadcast. Usually I pay only fleeting interest to these things, protected as I am from their impact by the comforts of modern life, like central heating and gritted roads. 'I think it might snow,' I had said, as I walked into the office.

No one appeared to take any notice. Instead, they seemed gripped by panic. Joy was busy sorting through boxes ('If I break another bloody nail, I'm going to sue,' she said repeatedly) while Kevin and Haley stood huddled round a list.

'There aren't enough, I don't think,' said Haley, concerned.

'Well, as long as that group goes to the one by the community hall, it should be OK,' Kevin replied.

I wondered what all the fuss was about until Lynne walked past. 'Give us a hand getting the last of the boxes up, would you?' she said, as she heaved one past me.

'What's going on?' I had asked, blissfully unaware of what freezing weather means to those living on the streets.

'Severe weather warning,' said Lynne, as she went back downstairs towards the entrance. I followed her. We went into the basement and there, among a few broken chairs and bits of old office furniture, were the boxes. Each contained army-issue sleeping-bags that would withstand temperatures of minus twenty degrees. Then she explained that, in weather like this, those sleeping out on the streets and exposed to the elements were at risk of literally freezing to death. I've never dreamt of a white Christmas since.

Upstairs, there was a frantic attempt, conducted with military precision by Kevin and Haley, to ensure that all our homeless patients had adequate shelter by the end of the day. While many were in hostels, a number slept in doorways or parks. Lynne had already gone on one trawl of the usual sleep-sites to round people up, but the nature of this group meant that they could be anywhere at any time. Joy had drawn up a rota so that each of us took it in turns to brave the icy weather searching for those who might have been missed. We handed out a schedule detailing pick-up points for minibuses, which had been chartered to take people to the various shelters. There was also a list of the shelters and what each offered. Some were in church halls, others in disused warehouses. Some allowed drinking. Most allowed dogs and even offered veterinary care. Doctors and dentists were on hand.

It occurred to me that until now I had been ignorant that each winter all this was going on. It was, quite literally, a matter of life and death for our patients. This sent a chill through me. Decisions that were made here in the office, just like in A&E Re-sus, had a direct bearing on whether or not someone would live. But in the clinical setting of the hospital, death is detached from everyday life. People come into hospital unwell and may or may not live. But doctors take off their stethoscopes and leave the hospital for the real world where the prospect of death does not loom large. Here, however, it cast its shadow over everyday public places. While Ruby had to deal with life-and-death decisions in the confines of Re-sus, here they were everywhere and boundless.

It was some time after all this that I remembered Patrick hadn't come back for his appointment. At first I thought nothing of it as I was used to people not attending. But as the day progressed, I began to worry. It seemed strange that someone so desperate and alone, who had made such an effort to come in the day before, would not return, especially when he knew we were trying to find him somewhere permanent to stay. I mentioned it to Lynne as she was unpacking more sleeping-bags, thinking she'd tell me not to be silly, but she didn't. 'You're sure he made it to the shelter last night?' she asked.

'I don't know,' I replied uneasily.

'It was minus four last night,' she said.

I waited for Patrick to appear that day and stayed well into the evening in case he came, but he didn't. On my way home I looked at everyone I passed, hoping to see him. I didn't.

Sitting at home round the kitchen table I told Ruby and Flora about him. 'You don't mean to tell me people actually sleep outside in this?' Flora said, horrified.

It was the following morning, as we all sat in the office, that Lynne warned me he might not have survived. Haley, always practical, had phoned round as many of the shelters as she could think of, making enquiries. 'I'll try the last one,' she said, as she picked up the phone.

Lynne smiled at me. 'There's nothing else we can do,' she said.

We sat there, trying not to listen to Haley's conversation. Even Joy had been upset that morning. She'd asked about Patrick almost as soon as she had walked in the door (well, after checking her hair, eating a croissant and applying lavish quantities of lipstick while sat at her desk). Haley put down the phone and shook her head. He wasn't there either. 'We'll check with the police again, but I'm afraid that's about all we can do,' she said.

'Is it worth going out for a look?' I asked.

'You can if you want to,' said Lynne. 'I don't think it'll do any good, and perhaps ...' She stopped as she tried to find a kind way to phrase it. 'There are lots of other people who could do with your help. Perhaps we should focus on them today.'

She was probably right. I stood up. 'I should go to the hostel,' I said. 'Warren called yesterday. A few of the men have chest infections and I should check they don't turn into pneumonia.'

'You never know,' said Kevin, trying to be chipper, 'miracles do happen.' He nibbled his biscuit, looking, I thought, remarkably like a chipmunk. Lynne glared at him although I wasn't sure if this was because she disapproved of him giving me false hope or because he was making crumbs.

'What about Barry?' I asked, knowing that he regularly slept in the open.

'He's usually good at sorting himself out,' said Lynne. I was still worried. I had felt indebted to him ever since the night he'd saved my life, and felt frustrated that I'd had no way of repaying his bravery. I had thanked him, but I always got the impression that words meant nothing to Barry: they were like distant murmurings he could hear but not understand. Likewise, there was nothing material I could give him that would articulate to him how I felt as he had no interest in possessions. 'I'll try to find him after I go to the hostel,' I said.

Professor Pierce stood up. 'Well, I must be off. I have a meeting. But do keep me abreast of any developments.' He gave me a little nod as he walked past.

'Try not to worry too much, darling,' said Joy. 'You did everything you could – and maybe Kevin's right. You never know, perhaps he'll have found somewhere else to stay so he's all right. And if you pass anywhere that sells Hobnobs . . .'

I knew that if Patrick hadn't gone to the hostel after I'd seen him, something must have happened. He'd have tried to sleep out one more night, the cold would have got to him and . . . It didn't bear thinking about. I picked up my bag and coat, walked down the stairs and out into the bitterly cold morning. Professor Pierce was ahead of me, down the road. He worked at the Phoenix Project part time; the rest he spent as an academic. It was a source of fascination to me how he had managed to combine two such polarised professions: on the one hand he worked in the rarefied environs of the university, writing books and doing research, lecturing bright young things who had known only privilege and comfort, while on the other he mixed with the most disenfranchised and dishevelled groups in society.

'You need a bit of a mix,' he had once said, when I'd asked him about it. He was my boss and had wanted to know what had happened with Barry on the night when he had saved my life. We had met in his study at the university where he worked. It was small and poky and the one window looked out on to air-conditioning units, which rattled constantly. 'Working with the homeless is a privilege,' he had said. I looked at him, surprised. 'You see people at their rawest, their most

vulnerable, and it gives you an appreciation of the
fragility of the human condition.' He sat back in his
chair and put his hands on his stomach. 'As humans we
walk around in a state of perpetual delusion, believing
that ours is the only way of experiencing the world and
applying this to everything we encounter. As a result,
when we're challenged by things we can't understand,
that are different from or alien to us we're scared.' He
spoke slowly, as if selecting each word with great care.
He reached into the drawer as he spoke and produced
a box. 'What the patients in our line of work teach us
is that, despite our differences, we are all the same.
We have the same desires, motivations and concerns.
They teach us what it is to be human and it's always
a privilege to be taught,' he said. He opened the box
and produced a cigar. 'Do you smoke?' he said. I shook
my head. I didn't like cigars and reasoned it would be
gauche to produce my cigarettes.

He fumbled with the cigar for a few moments
before lighting it. This made me slightly anxious.
Surely he wasn't allowed to smoke in here. I looked
around, half expecting an official to appear and fine
him. None did, and I could see, from the nicotine
stains on the ceiling above his desk, that this was
not a concern that preoccupied him. He leant
forward and opened the window slightly. The noise
from the air-conditioning units briefly filled the
room before the window slid shut again. He paid it
no attention. 'Man cannot bear too much reality,'
he said. 'I often think that can be applied to our
patients, those who have run away, dipped out of
society, become alcoholics or drug-users. They do

it to avoid the reality of their lives.' He puffed at the cigar and held the smoke in his mouth for a few moments. 'It also applies to us. We have to be careful that, working in this field, we don't burn out. Things can sometimes be too . . .' he paused '. . . real. Be critical, thoughtful and reflexive, but don't become cynical, and never fall into the trap of judging because that closes off the mind. That's why I work in academia. It provides the light to the shade.' Piles of books covered nearly every surface. He picked one up, then put it down again. 'Did I offer you one?' he said, pushing the cigars forward.

'Yes, and no thanks. I'm fine, thank you,' I replied. So that was his secret, I thought. That was how he managed to do the job he did. Just as Amy had her strategy, her way of getting job satisfaction, so did Professor Pierce.

Now Professor Pierce went towards the station. I crossed the road and made my way to the hostel. People scurried past, wrapped up warmly against the biting cold. My nose was running and my ears burnt as the wind whipped about me. It was at times like this that I wished I'd listened to my mum and worn a thermal vest. I arrived at the hostel and stood in the entrance, shivering, for a few moments.

Warren the Warden approached, smiling. 'We've got a long list for you today,' he said. 'This weather, it's had them dropping like flies. Everyone's come down with flu.' Several men in the lobby smiled and waved, then resumed their conversations. Talcott whizzed past on his way out, calling hello.

Warren took me to my patients. Most had chest infections or 'flu. A few had HIV and needed more urgent treatment as a chest infection could develop rapidly into a more life-threatening condition.
It seemed a never-ending stream of people but, eventually, I finished. 'There's a new chap you should have a look at too,' said Warren, as I got up to leave after my last patient. He led me down the corridor and pushed open the door to one of the rooms. Inside a man was sitting on the bed. 'This is George,' said Warren to me. 'George, this is the doctor. Remember I said I thought it might be a good idea to talk to him?'

Warren turned to go and, as he passed me, grimaced. 'He's very depressed,' he whispered.

George had been homeless for two years but had slept on a friend's floor for the past year. When the friend had got a new girlfriend, George had felt increasingly unwelcome so he had left. He'd slept rough until he'd got a room at the hostel a few weeks ago. He made his money from begging and spent the rest of the time sitting in his room alone. 'I just don't see the point,' he said. He was certainly depressed. 'I'm never going to get a job, and if I can't get a job, I can't get out of here.'

This wasn't entirely true. There were adult-education schemes, training placements, but I could appreciate how, from his perspective, there must have appeared no way out. It takes motivation and determination to attend courses, and the hostel, with its grim paintwork and cold, echoey corridor, was unremittingly bleak. For some people this might be the source of their motivation, making them determined to get away, but when you're depressed to start with and find yourself in a place like this, it's hard to hold on to any hope that things might get better.

In the past he had used alcohol heavily but had stopped when he moved in with his friend. Since his arrival in the hostel, though, he had begun drinking again. 'Alcohol is a depressant. It'll only make you feel worse in the long run,' I said.

He tightened the sides of his mouth as he grappled with this awkward truth. 'I know,' he began. 'It's just that drinking's easy.'

He needed anti-depressants but ideally he'd have to stop drinking before I prescribed them. Looking round his miserable room, I wasn't sure that the environment was conducive to this. Also, I suspected there wasn't a tablet I could prescribe that would make everything better for George.

He had been happiest in the army. He hadn't liked school and had left at the age of sixteen with only a couple of O levels. After this he had spent several months helping his older brother clean carpets. He drifted aimlessly until, a year later, he and a friend decided to sign up. Suddenly his life had purpose. He had loved the discipline and routine, and went on campaigns all over the world. The army had provided him with a structure that his life had lacked. But when he had left to return to civilian life, things had never worked out for him. There had been no big event, no hideous trauma. He just couldn't adjust to life on Civvy Street. He had wandered aimlessly through life until, without work and drinking heavily, he found himself homeless.

There were lots of ex-servicemen on the streets. It seemed that most had been so used to the discipline of military life that when this was taken away they were left dazed and confused, bereft of any sense of belonging. Perhaps they would have been like this even if they hadn't joined the services, and the army had provided George with brief respite. But I wondered how you could be expected to cope in the real world if, from the age of sixteen, everything had been so rigidly controlled: you were trained to obey orders, to do precisely as you were told – in essence, to be institutionalised.

'If you can stay off the booze for a bit, we can give you anti-depressants to improve your mood.'

He looked momentarily hopeful. 'Do you think they'll work?' he asked, resting his head on his hand.

'I hope so,' I said before turning and leaving him alone in his room.

I left the hostel and made my way back to the office. Patrick was still on my mind and I found myself praying for a miracle.

'Freeze the bollocks off a brass monkey.'

I knew who it was before I looked up. 'Hello, Molly,' I said, smiling.

'Bloody 'ell, you don't wanna be out in this,' she said, moving into a doorway for shelter. She was pulling along her shopping trolley.

'I've been to see some patients and I'm heading back now. You just been for your methadone?'

'Yeah. Bloody 'ell, though, I nearly didn't come out, it was so cold. My front step was solid ice this mornin'.

I coulda snapped my neck if I'd stepped on it.' She dug her hands deep into her pockets. 'I saw you from right up the road. I knew it was you. I thought, either it's a crack-head, or it's that doctor.'

I was a little puzzled. I'd never been confused with a crack-head before.

'Yeah, everyone's noticed it. You got a crack walk.'

'A what?' I said.

'Crack walk,' she repeated. 'You know, you walk like someone who uses crack. You walk so fast and determined. It's a crack walk.'

I'd never heard of this, although I had often been on the streets and seen dishevelled patients race past with a strange fixed fervour.

'Yer crack users, they walk fast, head up, kinda wagglin' their hips as though they're about to break into a run.' She sucked her teeth. 'Yer heroin addicts, though, they gotta different walk. It's slower, still determined, but by the time they come to buy drugs, they're usually withdrawing so they're in a bit of pain and it shows in the way they put their feet down.'

This was brilliant. She was like the drug world's Desmond Morris.

'You walk like a crack addict,' she concluded.

I protested that it was because I was always oversleeping and in constant fear of Sister Stein's stick if I was late. 'And what type of walk do you have, then?' I asked jokingly.

'I walk like an eighty-year-old woman with a knackered hip, as well you know, you cheeky sod,' she said, laughing.

I walked back up the main road but detoured

momentarily to some of the regular sleep-sites I knew people used, partly to check that everyone had gone into a shelter, partly to see if I could find Patrick. Everywhere was deserted, and I breathed a sigh of relief. Walking by the bus shelters, though, I spied Barry and went up to him. 'You all right, Barry?' I asked. He had paper tied round his feet.

'Yes,' he replied, in his usual monotone.

'It's getting very cold and there've been severe-weather warnings. Don't you want to go somewhere warm?' I said. I explained about all the different shelters he could go to, and that he wouldn't have to stay long if he didn't want to. He shrugged. I wondered how long he'd be able to keep this sort of life up before he succumbed to the elements.

'We'd be very worried to think of you sleeping outside,' I said, 'and my mum would have kittens if she knew you were sitting out here in the freezing cold.' He shrugged again, but looked at me. 'I could let you have the address of the nearest one. There's even a minibus to take you.'

He paused for a moment. 'OK, then,' he said flatly.

I smiled. 'Just until the weather improves.' He nodded, and I handed him the address, then turned to walk away.

'Thank you,' he said suddenly.

'A pleasure,' I replied.

As I made my way past the station, I decided to pop into the supermarket on the concourse to get something to eat. In fact, I went with the explicit intention of consuming my body weight in yum-yums. Now, whoever invented the finger-long twists of sugar-coated dough, they couldn't have thought up a more appropriate name. They are what their name suggests. When God sent manna from heaven – and you might be hard pushed to find this in the Book of Exodus – it was surely in the form of yum-yums. Pure ambrosia, no question about it. I know that, as a doctor, I should be advocating organic dried fruit and nuts, but I was having a hard day: I was cold, miserable and I'd just been told I walked like a crack addict.

Tamsin was sitting by the doorway. She was one of Haley's patients whom I'd seen several times when I visited the hostel where she lived. 'Hello,' I said, in a voice that suggested I was a man on a yum-yum mission who didn't have time for idle chit-chat.

'Oh, hello, Dr Max,' she replied from the pavement. 'I don't like to ask, but you wouldn't by any chance, you know . . .' She trailed off, embarrassed. Then, 'You wouldn't have some spare change for food, would you, Doctor?' she blurted out.

The decision as to whether or not to give money to homeless people is fraught with difficulty, and although I'd worked with them for so long, I hadn't come to any conclusion as to the best way to help them. But, I reasoned, buying hungry people food isn't complex and I couldn't walk in there, buy myself something and go back out past her. She had schizophrenia and was hungry. I offered to buy her a sandwich. I'd get her a yum-yum too, I thought. I'm a great believer in the ameliorative power of yum-yums.

I knew, of course, that her problems wouldn't easily

be solved. The word 'homeless', unlike yum-yum, isn't a straightforward description. It doesn't just mean that you don't have a home. In a staggering number of cases, it also means you have a mental illness. So much for care in the community. While the large asylums of years ago were far from ideal, I wonder if living hand-to-mouth on the streets is progress.

Salivating at the prospect of the delights awaiting me as I entered the food aisles, I was rather surprised to find one of the assistants putting the store's entire yum-yum stock in a clear plastic bag. Sacrilege. I sidled up to her. 'What are you doing with the yum-yums?' I asked, trying hard to sound mature and authoritative.

'Well, they go out of date tomorrow,' was the reply.

'But it's today, not tomorrow,' I said.

'Yes, but we're clearing the shelves.'

It was then that a horrific realisation came over me. 'What are you going to do with all that food?' I asked.

'We bin it,' she said breezily, tossing some cheese and broccoli quiches into her rubbish bag.

I could see Tamsin's back against the glass while people streamed past her. She was hungry, and all this food was going to waste. 'Why not give some to the homeless people, like that girl outside?' I asked.

'We can't do that. If they ate it, and then got sick, they might sue.'

I didn't like to point out that they were without the money for a cup of tea, which made it unlikely they would launch a legal battle in the further unlikely event they were poisoned by a yum-yum. The stupidity of the situation was almost unbelievable: if I'd been five minutes earlier I'd have been able to pick the exact same food off the shelf that was apparently no longer fit for consumption and purchase it. While many supermarkets donate food within its use-by date to charity, a vast amount is thrown away. I stood there, powerless, while shelves of perfectly edible goods were cleared and people sat outside, begging for something to eat. Sometimes, it doesn't take a psychiatrist to see that the world's gone mad.

I returned to the office and was met by a row of eager faces. 'What?' I said, as I looked at them suspiciously.

Their smiles broke into grins. 'He's here.'

'Who?' I asked.

'Patrick. He's downstairs. And has he got a story to tell you, darling!' said Joy.

I was overwhelmed with relief, and when I went downstairs I almost kissed him. I didn't, of course, just shook his hand and chastised him for not turning up to my appointment the day before. 'What happened to you? We were all sick with worry,' I scolded. He sat down and told me about the last few days. Before that moment, I would not have believed that Patrick, a damaged and unloved ex-convict, would reaffirm my faith in humanity. But he did.

After his first meeting with me, he had walked along the road, trying to find his way to the shelter I had circled for him. What I had failed to realise, and Patrick had been too ashamed to tell me on our first meeting, was that he couldn't read. The address, the directions, the road signs meant nothing to him and, wandering around, he soon became confused and disoriented. He remembered the name of the road I had told him and asked passers-by for directions. When he got there, though, he couldn't find the shelter and realised there was probably more than one road with that name. He looked in his pocket and discovered he had lost the sheet I had given him so had no way of contacting us to ask for help. He set out again, trying to remember his way back, but became increasingly lost. He had been walking for nearly four hours in the freezing cold and it was getting dark. He was scared and alone and didn't know what to do.

It was then that he had met Mrs Clarence. She had been walking past and he had stopped her, explained that he was lost and asked if she knew where the shelter was. It was then that something amazing happened. Standing in the middle of the street, her arms weighed down with shopping bags, she didn't walk past him. She stood and talked to him. She explained that the only other road she knew of by that name was in the opposite direction and far away. Then, in a breathtaking act of compassion, she invited him to stay at her house for the night.

Patrick told the story in an incredulous tone, a wide smile across his face, and I suspected that this was the first time anyone had ever shown him kindness. He went home with her and had dinner with her and her husband. They didn't ask him about his past life, just what his plans were. He was so tired that he went to sleep straight after the meal. The next morning he came down and sat at the breakfast table. Mrs Clarence cooked him eggs, then explained that she and her husband had made some phone calls. She had spoken to some of the congregation at the church where they went and they wanted to help. The vicar had said he could sleep in the church until the bad weather passed, and he could pay his way by doing odd jobs. Mrs Clarence gave him one of her husband's coats, a pair of gloves and a scarf, and drove him to the church. There, he met the vicar and the person who arranged the flowers, and they talked to him and made him tea. That night he had slept in the vestry.

The following morning Mrs Clarence had come to see him. She had found the address of the Phoenix Project and told him he should come and see me and tell me everything was all right. She had given him the bus fare, shown him where to go, and here he was. He went back to the church that night and stayed there for several weeks. The congregation sort of adopted him, and the last I heard someone was teaching him to read, and they had found him a job helping on a fruit-and-veg stall.

There is a beautiful passage in the Book of Hebrews that begins, 'Let us show hospitality to strangers, for in doing so some have entertained angels unawares.' Patrick was no angel, I'm convinced of that, but Mrs Clarence had faith in humanity. She didn't know him and she took a chance. Perhaps what she did was foolish and naïve, and if things had turned out differently, this might have been a story about how we shouldn't trust anyone, just walk on by when someone needs our help.

But she had taken a chance. I'm pleased she did. If she hadn't, he might be dead. And she made me think that perhaps there were angels out there, after all.

Chapter 14

'You owe me forty quid,' growled the man, as I opened the door to the women's hostel.

Erm, no, I certainly do not, I thought. But, as his fists were the size of my head, I smiled benignly and cleared my throat. 'Sorry, can I help you?' I replied tentatively, preparing to slam the door in his face and hide under a table.

I was feigning ignorance: I knew exactly why he had knocked on the door. From down the corridor of the hostel I could hear Jeanette shouting, 'I told you not to open the door. You're gonna get us killed!'

I'd only come to prescribe her some medication and have a chat, and now look at the mess I was embroiled in.

'Tell 'im to eff off,' she screamed.

Erm, maybe you'd like to do that yourself. After all, you got us into this situation in the first place.

'Look, mate,' I began, in my most cringeworthy mockney accent, through the crack in the door, and quickly realised that wasn't the tack to take.

'I ain't your mate,' he told me.

That was very true. It worked for Jamie Oliver, though. I cleared my throat. I'll try the posh approach,

I thought, and got ready with my Prince Charles impression. Just then the man lunged for me and tried to push past. I slammed the door as hard and fast as I could. Phew. At times like that, social etiquette had to go out of the window and so, it seemed, had Jeanette. 'What are you doing?' I called after her, as she clambered out of the back window.

'I'm gettin' out of 'ere,' she yelled.

What did she know that I didn't? 'Why? You can't just leave. I'm in the middle of telling you the importance of regular health screening.'

'It'll be you that needs health screening if you stay in there,' she said, now dangling precariously off the window-ledge. 'He thinks you're my pimp. He won't give up. Trust me, they never do. Best to scarper while you can still use your legs.'

Me? A pimp? I'm all for equal opportunities in the workplace but, really, as if I'd ever get a job as a pimp.

I looked back at the door, which the man was now hitting at regular intervals. Not my face, please, not that, I thought. There was only one thing for it. 'I can't believe I'm doing this,' I said, as I ran to the back room and swung my leg over the windowsill. Jeanette had already dropped to the ground below.

'Just be grateful we ain't on the third floor,' she said.

That's right: always look on the bright side. I'd almost forgotten to do that, amid the fear of being murdered by a man twice the size of a bus with half its IQ. I held on to the window-ledge and dropped down. Thud. I stood up. Ta-da! No bones broken. But Jeanette was already clambering over the fence. 'Oh, no, I draw the line at that.' I put my hands on my hips and stood firm. 'This is ridiculous.' I hadn't gone to medical school for six years so that I could shimmy up drainpipes and pole-vault over fences.

'Fine. Stay there if you want,' she said.

The man appeared at the open window. 'Give me what I paid for!'

I took my hands off my hips and swallowed. I gave him a little wave. 'Hello again,' I said. About ten seconds later, it became apparent that, should I ever wish to leave medicine, a promising career in the hundred-metre hurdles was a definite option. 'He's coming after us,' I bellowed, as I cleared the fence and hit the ground running.

All this was about 'clipping'. Before I'd started my job, I'd had no idea what it meant. In a horribly middle-class moment, when Jeanette explained that this was how she made her money, I assumed it had something to do with the *Cutty Sark*. How strange, I had thought, that a homeless drug addict with schizophrenia should be involved in tea importing. Actually, it's about prostitution. Clipping is the slang term for when a prostitute is paid for a service up-front, then does a runner rather than carrying it out. To my mind, men paying for sex don't have a moral leg to stand on when they find themselves the victim of such a crime. The greater crime is sleeping with a vulnerable, mentally ill woman. If anyone is a victim, surely it's her. It's a complicated moral landscape and I'm not going to make excuses for Jeanette's lifestyle – not least because, thanks to her, I was being chased by a sex-starved maniac. But she couldn't easily change her situation and perhaps she was in that situation because her choices had been taken away from her. She used drugs because they gave short symptomatic relief from her schizophrenia, although of course in the long term they made it worse. One of the strange things about crack is that it induces people who don't hear voices to hear them, and in those who do hear voices, it makes them go away. Only temporarily, of course: they come back, more insistent, shortly afterwards. The sufferer begins a downward spiral, using crack to stop the voices and having to take it more and more frequently.

To fund this lifestyle Jeanette was a prostitute. Her activities had gained her an ASBO although, in my opinion, the men were far more anti-social than she was. Jeanette's behaviour was driven by need: more ante-social than anti-social. Dozens of my patients had ASBOs. They'd got them for doing things that were motivated by the need to survive, like begging and prostitution. The courts might as well not have bothered: people like Jeanette weren't going to stop what they were doing just because they had a bit of paper from a judge telling them to.

On the other side of the fence, I discovered, to my horror, that a driveway with a locked gate led to the main road. I sighed. Why hadn't I taken the leafy-suburb job with the nice old ladies and a guaranteed income of Quality Street as Ruby had suggested? Jeanette was already halfway up the gate. She had clearly done this before. The man was now attempting to scale the fence and continued to demand, at full volume, his money back or the services promised to him, despite my assurances that I was most certainly not going to provide him with either, especially not the latter if the size of his hands where anything to go by.

On the other side of the fence, the grass was indeed greener – the danger of being mauled by the maniac had gone. The fence was too high for him and we left him shouting on the other side. The whole encounter had been rather reminiscent of a Benny Hill sketch, I thought, as we walked away and chuckled to myself. I'm going to miss all this when I go back to life on the wards. Suddenly Jeanette sprinted off. 'Run!' she screamed. I turned just in time to see the man land on the other side of the fence. He saw my face. We stared at each other. I smiled and gave a little wave, then took to my heels. Miss this? Who was I kidding?

I arrived at the drug-dependency unit out of breath and flustered. 'You all right?' said Tony, as I took refuge in the office.

'Fine. I've just been mistaken for a pimp and pursued across half of the city by a sex-starved meat-head. All in a day's work.'

Tony shrugged. 'Horses for courses, mate,' he said. 'Except you're not–'

'I know,' I interrupted.

Bruce looked up: 'Exit, pursued by a bear,' he said.

Tony looked at him. 'Yeah, except he just told us it was a man who chased him, not a bear.'

'*The Winter's Tale*, Act Three, scene three,' said Bruce.

It wasn't the patients who posed a risk to my mental health; it was most definitely the staff. I left the office.

In the waiting room I found Fergal and Anthony, who gave me their usual cheeky grins. 'OK, who's first?' I said.

Fergal stood up and followed me into the interview room. 'Doctor,' he said, as we sat down. He was looking at me strangely.

'Yes?' I said warily, suspecting he was about to tell me something I didn't want to hear. I looked down at his prescription form and saw that both he and Anthony were on tiny amounts of methadone and it could be stopped altogether in a few weeks. They had managed not to use heroin for months. I knew he was about to tell me they had relapsed.

'You know that form you filled out for us for Social Services?' he said.

'Yes,' I replied, still anxious about what he was going to tell me.

He bit his bottom lip. 'They've given us a room each in a hostel and put us on the housing list.'

I blinked. 'You haven't used any heroin?'

'No,' said Fergal, taken aback. 'We've stopped doing that now. We're clean. We're never going back to that life. It sucked,' he said proudly.

I smiled at him. My success story, I thought. And, out of all my patients, those two were the ones I'd been convinced would fail. They'd proved me wrong and I couldn't have been happier.

Now the next chapter of their lives was opening and I felt excited for them. OK, so they weren't about to take up jobs as merchant bankers and move into a penthouse overlooking the river. Perhaps living in a hostel and not injecting drugs was a small step to getting their lives back on track but it was a start and it represented an enormous change in how they viewed themselves.

There was potential, I thought, as I listened to Fergal tell me about the plans he and Anthony had. I wondered what role I had played in all this. Had I said something that had clicked and started a chain reaction that had ended in them being drug-free? Had I played a part in their transformation, or had I been incidental to it? I didn't know how to ask this question without sounding like a glory-hunter. I resigned myself to the fact that I would never know. Perhaps Fergal and Anthony didn't know and maybe, for them, it didn't matter.

'I'm leaving at the end of the week so I probably won't see you again,' I said to Fergal, 'but . . .' I wasn't sure what to say, '. . . well done. You should be proud of yourselves.'

He smiled, 'Thank you,' and held out his hand.

'It's true, you should both be proud of yourselves. It's a great achievement what you've done.'

Fergal shook his head. 'No, I meant thank you. Thank you for believing we could do it.' He got up to go, still proffering his hand. I shook it, but felt suddenly guilty that, actually, I hadn't believed in them. Amy had been right: you could get satisfaction from knowing you were making things a little bit less of a mess. But nothing could beat the feeling I'd had as I'd sat with Fergal. Unlike Ruby's line of work, it might not have made for a riveting episode of *ER*, and the rewards were more haphazard and not as instant, but it was just as worthwhile. I followed Fergal outside and he sat down next to Anthony. I looked at them both. My five per cent, I thought, and smiled.

It would be unfair to leave you with the impression that all was well at the drug-dependency unit. It was not. While Fergal and Anthony had shown me that it was possible to change, and that sometimes those you least expected to could prove you wrong, the converse was also true.

José sat in front of me. When I'd first met him, a successful, well-educated, intelligent man, I had thought he would be off heroin within a few weeks. That had been months ago. He'd made no real progress. 'Oh, you do not know what it is like,' he said, flicking his hand at me. 'I hate all this. I just want you to give me a pill and make it go away.'

I shook my head. 'You're still smoking heroin,' I said. 'Nothing is going to change until you stop using it.'

'Bah!' he said, widening his eyes. 'You don't understand. Without the heroin I can't sleep after coke and I need my sleep.' We had this conversation every time I saw José. It was pointless repeating myself, I reasoned. He knew as well as I did that he had to stop using cocaine, but he couldn't see how the two drugs were linked for him.

'It's not fair,' he began. 'All my friends use coke and they're not addicted to heroin.'

'Yes,' I replied, 'but now that your body has got used to relying on heroin to sleep after you've used cocaine, you won't be able to cut one out without stopping the other.'

He sat back in his chair with a sigh. 'And besides,' he added, 'I have to stop the heroin because I have a new boyfriend. He would freak if he knew I took heroin.'

'Well, that's a good motivation for you. What does he do?'

'He a fashion designer too,' he replied sulkily.

'Does he use cocaine?' I asked, knowing how difficult it is to stop if you're in a relationship with someone who uses.

José shook his head. 'No, he not approve of drugs.'

It took a few moments for the implication of this to sink in. 'Hang on,' I said, remembering what José had said when we'd first met. 'You told me you used coke because everyone in fashion did.' José nodded, oblivious. 'Well, you've just said your boyfriend doesn't yet he works in fashion.' José shifted in his seat. 'So clearly that's not true. If your boyfriend can manage without cocaine, why can't you?'

José couldn't answer this. 'He's different to me,' he said, flustered.

I was afraid that José would have to be the next doctor's project. He had built up a justification for his use of drugs and it would take time for him to see that it was not based in reality. But at least he had been confronted with this. That, I supposed, was progress of a sort.

Likewise Janice was having a difficult time. To her credit she had managed to stop using the over-the-counter painkillers. But when we had tried to reduce the methadone she had not coped well. Her dose had only been reduced a small amount and she had not experienced withdrawal symptoms, but she had come back the following week and insisted we increase the dose. She had begun to experience panic attacks at the thought of it being reduced any further. It was almost as if she needed to be addicted to something – like an alcoholic who becomes sober, then turns into a workaholic. All I had done with her was to replace one addiction, to painkillers, with another, to methadone. Clearly her addiction was performing some deep-seated psychological function. Maybe it gave her a purpose in life, something to structure it round, something definite and immovable, and the prospect of change frightened her too much. But at least methadone didn't consume her life in the way that obtaining painkillers had. Her husband still didn't know about her 'silliness' and I wondered if he ever would.

On my last day at the clinic, because she was now stable, I offered to change her from weekly to fortnightly prescriptions. She would have none of that. 'Oh, no,' she said. 'I quite like coming here. I've grown to enjoy sitting in the waiting room.' She chatted to the other patients and had made a number of friends over the months. 'It makes a change from the ladies I meet at bridge,' she said, with a laugh. 'Some of the patients are such characters, aren't they? You could write a book about them.'

'You could indeed,' I agreed, grinning.

I had seen so many people over the year, and so many had started treatment but dropped out. They had failed to turn up for appointments, left prescriptions uncollected, and had faded back whence they had come. Sometimes I wondered what had happened to them. 'They'll be back when they're ready,' Sister Stein promised, but by then I'd be long gone.

Georgia was still in hospital after the fiasco a month ago but, no doubt, would continue to use crack when she was discharged. Tammy, whom I'd been so determined to cure when I'd first met her, was a minor success. She had stopped injecting heroin and smoked it infrequently now, usually when she bumped into an old dealer; Sister Stein assured me this was an achievement. Amy had found out about further education for her, and now that heroin no longer dominated her life, she was thinking of doing a beauty-therapy course.

Then, of course, there was Molly. Sometimes a city can be large and anonymous, but after a chance encounter it can seem small and as though our lives are interconnected. I met Molly once more, a few months into my next job. It might surprise you to learn that she had given up drugs, although not out of choice. I was working in dementia care and was visiting a patient in a nursing home. I walked in, glanced into the sitting room and there, watching television, was Molly. She had had a fall at home, then a minor stroke, which had meant she could no longer look after herself. In a nursing home she couldn't get hold of heroin so she was on regular methadone. The stroke had affected her memory so although she recognised me, she couldn't place me. But, as Tony might say, a leopard doesn't change its spots and she was still 'effin and blindin' as she always had. Not, of course, that she was a leopard, as Tony would also feel obliged to point out.

I never found out what happened to Rachel's baby and, to be honest, I didn't want to. Some stories are better left unfinished.

It was perhaps fitting that one of the last patients I saw at the drug-dependency unit was cured before she even walked through the door. I like to count her as one of my five per cent, although her success had nothing to do with me.

Petra was thirty and a prostitute. She had been injecting a bag of heroin a day for the past eight years. She rolled up her sleeves and showed me her pockmarked arms. 'I was also injecting into my legs,' she said. Many patients had resorted to this: a vein might last, if you were lucky, a year or two, but eventually it collapsed and was useless. The longer someone injected, the more adventurous they had to be with finding a suitable vein. Injecting into the top of the legs, though, was particularly dangerous. The artery, where the blood was under considerable pressure, ran right next to the vein. People had been known to puncture it instead of the vein and haemorrhage to death. It also carried the risk of infection travelling up and into the spine, resulting in paralysis. Others got thromboses and had to have their legs amputated.

I was confused as to why Petra had come, though. 'But you don't use drugs any more?' I asked.

'No,' she said proudly. 'I've been clean for over a month.'

'So why are you here?' I asked. 'You don't need any more treatment.'

'Well, I haven't seen a doctor and I thought I should get checked out.'

'What about the doctor who treated you?' I asked.

'I treated myself,' she replied. 'I decided I'd had enough of drugs so I went to a friend's farm in Spain.'

'But how did you get methadone?' I asked. 'Did someone in Spain prescribe it for you?'

She shook her head. 'I didn't use methadone. I just stopped.'

'What?' I was amazed. 'What about the withdrawals? They're supposed to be agonising.'

'Yes,' she said simply, 'they are. I thought I was going to die. But I decided I'd rather die trying to get clean than as a drug addict.'

Her friend had locked her into the barn each night with a bucket and nursed her during the day. It had taken a month for her to stop withdrawing. The pain all over her body had been excruciating, and for the first week she had had constant diarrhoea. There were, I thought, easier, less painful ways. But perhaps having gone through all that pain she would never be tempted to go back to drugs. It was also a salutary lesson in how, if you really wanted to stop, you could.

Back in the office it was time to say my goodbyes. I still had one more day to do at the Phoenix Project, but I had seen my last patient at the drug-dependency unit. I kissed Amy and Meredith goodbye and shook Tony's hand.

'"Parting is such sweet sorrow,"' said Bruce, getting up to shake my hand.

'*Romeo and Juliet*,' I said.

His jaw dropped. 'Yes,' he said slowly. 'Act Two, scene one.' He looked round the office at everyone. 'So, you've learnt something since you've been here,' he said proudly.

I didn't think it kind to tell him I'd done it for GCSE English Literature.

Last was Sister Stein. She had been such an important figure in my life for the past year but I wasn't expecting an emotional farewell from her, which was good because I didn't get one. 'Well done,' she said plainly.

I thanked her and made to leave.

'Don't I get a kiss?' she said indignantly.

I smiled and obliged. 'You know the patients call you the Cattle Prod?' I said, with a wink.

'Of course I do – and if you don't get out of here, you'll find out why,' she said, brandishing her stick. And with that, I left.

Chapter 15

It was my last day. I had no patients booked in to see me as Joy had saved them for the doctor replacing me. But I still had a few loose ends to tie up, and Professor Pierce had impressed on me the importance of saying goodbye to the patients: 'They've let you into their lives and it's important that they're allowed to let you out again,' he had said, then left, forgetting to say goodbye to me.

I wasn't sure how I'd go about tracking down all the patients I had seen, given that I could rarely find them when I wanted to. I spent the morning catching up on paperwork and clearing my desk. Tomorrow I would be working in a completely new environment, with different people, different patients and yet more to learn.

In the afternoon there were some people I wanted to check up on at the hostel and Lynne had said she would come with me. I went up to the office to say goodbye. We all stood there awkwardly for a few moments, promising to keep in touch – much as I had with the nurses at the end of my junior-doctor year. At that moment I was incredibly grateful to them all for everything they had taught me and the experiences we had shared, but I didn't know how to tell them so.

'Come on, pay up,' said Lynne, to Joy. Joy's face was like thunder.

'What's going on?' I asked.

No one answered, but Lynne stood there smiling and holding out her hand.

Joy huffed and ferreted through her bag. 'Here,' she said coldly. 'I'm blaming you for this,' she said, pointing at me. She brought out her purse, opened it and took out a five-pound note. Reluctantly she handed it to Lynne.

'We had a bet,' said Lynne, grinning, 'and Joy lost, didn't you, Joy?'

'All right, darling, don't rub it in,' she said through gritted teeth.

'Joy bet me you wouldn't last,' said Lynne, 'and I bet you would.'

'He nearly didn't. He was on the brink of leaving, I could tell,' Joy mumbled.

'Here you go,' said Lynne, handing me the fiver. 'You can use it to buy a tie for your next job. No grubby T-shirts for you any more.'

That hadn't even occurred to me, so accustomed had I grown to wearing whatever I found on the floor each morning and this being totally acceptable. In fact, the more creased the better. I put the note in my pocket and went to hug Joy.

'All right, easy,' she said, holding up her hands. 'I've had enough trouble growing these nails. If I break another and have to resort to acrylics again, there'll be trouble.' But she leant forward and gave me a loud kiss on the cheek. 'There,' she said, wiping the lipstick off my face with the side of her hand, 'even if you never did get me any Hobnobs and have just cost me a fiver.' I said goodbye to Haley and Kevin, who stood at the top of the stairs and waved me off.

'Meet you in the hostel in an hour or so,' Lynne called after me.

I walked down the road, through the park to some council flats. There was one person I couldn't leave without saying goodbye, even if at this moment he wasn't technically homeless: Mr Allsop. He was still convinced he was God but had, miraculously, kept taking his medication. He hadn't gone back to the streets and hadn't been back to hospital.

I knocked on the door and heard him shuffling up to open it. 'My child,' he exclaimed, when he saw my face.

'I can't stop. I just wanted to say goodbye. It's my last day.'

He held up a finger. 'Hang on,' he said, shuffled off and returned a few minutes later with a pebble. 'The word of the Lord,' he said, handing it to me.

'Erm, thanks,' I said, smiling. Yep, still completely mad.

At the men's hostel, Lynne was waiting for me outside and we went in together. Talcott was sitting on his skateboard in the lobby. 'Have you still not got a glass eye?' I asked him, annoyed that although I'd filled in endless referral forms for him to have one fitted he still had an empty socket. 'And, come to think of it, what about your wheelchair? I asked for that months ago,' I said.

Talcott grinned toothily. 'Yeah, I got them,' he said, 'and the wheelchair's OK but it's not as good as my skateboard.'

'But what about the glass eye?' I asked.

'Well, I don't make so much money begging with it in, so I take it out when I go out and pop it back when I come home. The lads have started calling me Popeye.' I shook my head disapprovingly and Lynne laughed. I went and saw as many of the patients I could to say goodbye.

I hadn't been able to find Barry to say goodbye to him. Maybe it wouldn't have meant anything to him anyway, but part of me wanted to think that it would. I still have that Prada shirt and sometimes I wear it. I never admit to anyone how I came by it.

Lynne and I walked together to the main road. She was going back to the office and I was going home. We hugged. 'Thanks for everything,' I said.

'Don't forget us,' she called after me.

I walked back down the street, reflecting on the past year. I had started that job with questions I wanted answered. I had wanted to know why people ended up on the streets or using drugs. I had heard lots of stories, but I still couldn't answer the question. I had realised, though, that no single thing could be blamed; no single absolute causative factor stood out.

It occurred to me then that the question had been too simple and had failed to take into account that the things I had been looking at were symptoms of wider problems. There was no single answer to solving homelessness or drug addiction because there was no single cause. That, I thought, was at least partly an answer, although maybe not the one I had hoped for.

I phoned Ruby. 'Fancy a drink?' I asked.

'Yeah, but I won't be done here for at least another hour or so. See you at home?'

'Sure. I'll phone Flora and see if she's up for it,' I suggested.

'Oh, yeah, and find out if Lewis will come and cook for us,' she added.

The two constants in my life: that kitchen table, and that Ruby would never be domesticated.

I continued to walk towards the station. Two men stood on the other side of the road. They waved at me and I waved back. As I walked further away from the Phoenix Project building, the crowds swelled on the pavements and I was no longer alone on the street. The urban decay fell away and the shops stopped selling cut-price telephone calls to Africa, laptops at knock-down prices and cheap clothing. Slowly, commuter affluence took hold. I approached the station.

'Spare any change?' said a voice, and I looked down. I hesitated for a moment.

'Hey, you that doctor from the Phoenix Project?' he said. 'It's Samuel, remember?'

I did. He was the man with the gangrenous leg I'd been with when someone had spat at me. He'd had an amputation. We chatted briefly.

'I don't suppose you've got any spare change?' he said.

I put my hand into my pocket and felt the five-pound note. I paused. 'Sure. Here you go,' I said, handing it to him.

'Cheers, Doc,' he said, then turned to another passer-by. 'Spare any change?'

Acknowledgements

I am very grateful to a number of people who helped and supported me while writing this book:

the staff at the *Daily Telegraph*, both past and present: Liz Hunt, Maria Fitzpatrick, Genevieve Fox, George Cover, Penny Cranford, Maria Trkulja, Becky Pugh, Paul Clements, Andrew Pierce, Glenda Cooper, Fiona Hardcastle, Chloe Rhodes, Richard Preston, Joyce Smith, Robert Colvile; Barney Calman and Sarah Hartley at the *Mail on Sunday*, and Sarah Sands and the staff at *Reader's Digest*. Sincere thanks to those at Hodder whose support and encouragement have been overwhelming: Lisa Highton, Heather Rainbow, Cecilia Moore, Jack Fogg and Henry Jeffreys. And warm thanks to Heather Holden-Brown and Elly James who have been, as always, wonderful.

Special thanks also to Tasha Coccia, Rhiannon Burton, Sarah McMahon, Anna Berridge, Marios Pierides, Ben, Becky and Harry Fisher, Ruth-Ellen Davies, Toby Commerford, Andrew Solomon and John Habich-Solmon, Sue McCartney-Snape, François Borne, Dr Katz, Dr Ellis, Dr Rands, Dr Davids, Dr Lewis, Dr Weisblatt, Dr Bhakshi, Dr Thompson, Prof Littewood,

Prof Bhugra, Margaret Sharpe, Jacob Freeman,
Tony Grew, Fernando Alves, Maureen Lipman, Amy
Rosenthal, Jill Leslie, Susie Kilshaw, Pete-John Graeger,
Nadine Banna, the Gardiners, Katharine Lynch, Beth
Mallum, Neil Kirsch, Dean Thorpe, Christine Webber
and David Delvin, Jan Moir and Chris Stevens.

And, of course, my mum and my grandparents.
Finally, not forgetting my goldfish, Daniel: OK,
so he didn't exactly support me, but he did look
appropriately encouraging when I stared into his bowl
wondering if I'd ever get this book finished.

Heroin used 70?